Arterial B.
Made Easy

MW00438940

Dr A. B. Anup
MBBS, MD (Int Med)
DB M, DBA (Manag - UK)
MRCP (Int Med - UK),
BCIM (Int Med - USA)

What will you learn from this book :

What are the various components of a blood gas report
How to use these components and their pitfalls
Step by step approach to interpreting a blood gas report
How to confirm the given blood gas report is correct
PaO2, SaO2, CaO2, Pulse oximetry
Answers to many more questions you always wanted to know
And much more

Disclaimer

Every effort has been made to
ensure that the information in
this book is as accurate and as
up to date as possible. However,
for the sake of simplicity some
topics are oversimplified. You
are recommended to consult a
text book for further explanations.

Neither the author, nor the publisher,
nor the editor can accept any legal
responsibility for an error or omission
that may have occurred.

First edition   June 1996
First reprint   September 1996

Published by : A B Anup

This book is likely to be useful to

- Any physician or surgeon taking care of patients with a respiratory problem
- Residents in medicine
- Critical care nurses, residents and fellows
- Respiratory care nurses, residents and fellows
- Respiratory therapists
- Third and fourth year medical students
- Medical students in the first and the second year to understand the respiratory physiology and pathology
- Anyone preparing for the NBME, USMLE, FLEX, PLAB, MRCP (UK) exam
- Physician assistants taking care of patients with respiratory problems
- Anyone dealing with intubated patients including anesthesiologists, intensivists, pulmologists and internists
- Paediatricians and Neonatologists

This book is especially written in simple English so that the maximum number of medical professionals in different countries can benefit from it.

How to Get The Most From This Book

Although there are books on the market concerning the Arterial Blood Gases (and some will come in the future), lack of a concise but comprehensive book on the subject has always been a complaint from my students. I have written this book to address that issue. I have tried to make it simple, short but comprehensive, easy to carry around and cheap to fit a resident's and student's budget.

At the outset I recommend that you throw away the ABG card as you will not be permitted to use it in the examination. Carry this book with you and refer it to as and when needed. Ultimately, learn to interpret all ABG reports without any outside help.

If you are a beginner start with chapter 1 and go chapter by chapter through the book. Before you go to section II you must read and understand section I. Even if you are a pro, I strongly recommend that you read section I in your free time.

If you like challenges in life - pick up a pencil and a paper and solve exercises A to G in section III. Each exercise (A,B,C...G) should take you less than six minutes to solve. That's how long it will take you once you have mastered this book. If you can complete section III in 45 minutes or less(without the help of the ABG graph) and score above 85 percent, you probably do not need to read this book. But, if not, I suggest you read it.

Clinically important points are highlighted and this will help when you revew for the exams.

My best wishes to you.

A B Anup, MD
September 10, 1996

CONTENTS

Abbreviations

ABG	=	Arterial blood gas
A-aDO$_2$	=	Alveolo-arterial oxygen gradient
BE	=	Base excess
CaO$_2$	=	Oxygen content of the whole blood
CHF	=	Congestive heart failure
CO	=	Carbon monoxide
CO$_2$	=	Carbon dioxide
COPD	=	Chronic obstructive pulmonary disease
Deoxy Hb	=	Deoxyhemoglobin (reduced hemoglobin)
FiO$_2$	=	Fraction of oxygen in inspired air/gas
H+	=	Hydrogen ion concentration
Hb	=	Hemoglobin
Hb-O$_2$	=	Hemoglobin Oxygen (dissociation curve)
HCO$_3$	=	Bicarbonate
O$_2$	=	Oxygen
Oxy Hb	=	Oxyhemoglobin
PaO$_2$	=	Partial pressure of oxygen in the arterial blood (Commonly, also called PO$_2$)
PAO2	=	Partial pressure of oxygen an the air in the alveolus
PaCO$_2$	=	Partial pressure of carbon dioxide in arterial blood (Commonly also called PaCO$_2$)
P$_B$	=	Barometric pressure or atmospheric pressure
PiO$_2$	=	Partial pressure of oxygen in the inspired air
PvO$_2$	=	Partial pressure of oxygen in the venous blood
pH	=	Negative logarithm of hydrogen ion concentration (indicates acidity or alkalinity of the medium)
SaO$_2$	=	Saturation of hemoglobin in the arterial blood
SpO$_2$	=	Saturation of hemoglobin in the peripheral blood (i.e. Capillary blood)
VBG	=	Venous blood gas
WVP	=	Water vapor pressure

Section 1

Basics of Blood Gas Analysis

Chapter 1 :   Introduction

How To Get Maximum Information From The Blood Gas Report

Following is a typical arterial blood gas report :

pH / $PaCO_2$ / PaO_2 / HCO_3 / BE / SaO_2

In a non- emergency situation make it a habit to read the ABG in the following manner. By following this sequence you are less likely to miss the unusual conditions and will be more confident in case of an emergency.

Always read a blood gas in context of the clinical picture of the patient :
As you will see in the following pages, each numerical value of a blood gas result has a limited significance if read on its own i.e. without knowing the clinical picture. This is because of the number of confounders and variables affecting each parameter of the report. Most institutions use instruments that give the ABG report printouts without the patients' names and therefore errors in ABG reporting do occur sometimes. (The author knows of incidences where patients were almost intubated as the wrong blood gas report was being ascribed to them). If the ABG report does not make sense, do not hesitate to repeat it or to get help from your seniors or colleagues. The implications of wrong treatment because of a wrong ABG report can be disastrous for the patient and may be difficult to correct later on.

READ WHAT IS OBVIOUS ON THE ABG REPORT :

Number 1 . SaO_2 (Saturation of the hemoglobin by oxygen)
Number 2 . HCO_3 and BE (Bicarbonate and Base Excess)
Number 3. PaO_2 (Partial pressure of O_2 in blood. Also called PO_2)
Number 4. $PaCO_2$ (Partial pressure of CO_2 in blood. Also called PCO_2)
Number 5. pH

READ WHAT IS NOT OBVIOUS ON THE ABG REPORT :

Number 6. $A-aDO_2$ (A-a gradient or alveoloarterial oxygen gradient).

Clinically, in an ABG report pH, $PaCO_2$, PaO_2 and $A-aDO_2$ are the most important parameters. This we will see in the following pages.

Chapter 2 : SaO$_2$ v / s PaO$_2$

SaO$_2$: Oxygen Saturation of the Hemoglobin :

Always compare SaO$_2$ with the PaO$_2$. Following are clinically important corresponding points :

PaO$_2$	SaO$_2$*	Clinical Importance
40	75	Normal venous PO$_2$ (PvO$_2$)
55	88	Indication for home oxygen therapy
59	89	Indication for home oxygen therapy in a COPD patient with complications e.g. CHF or polycythemia
60	90	Point where steep fall in partial pressure of oxygen in the plasma occurs. Every attempt must be made to maintain PaO$_2$ above this level to prevent tissue hypoxia
80	95	Lower end of normal range for PaO$_2$
100	97	Higher end of normal range for PaO$_2$
150	99	Theoretically maximum attainable PaO$_2$ breathing room air at sea level
159	99.9	Theoretically maximum attainable PaO$_2$ breathing dry room air (without any water vapor - see chapter on A-a gradient)

*This correlation is approximate only.

SaO$_2$ measures the percentage of hemoglobin in oxidized form and thus saturated with oxygen. Clinically, it is done by pulse oximetry (see below) where emitter and receiver probes are used to determine oxidized and reduced hemoglobins. **SaO$_2$ on the arterial blood gas is a calculated value derived from the PaO$_2$.**

PaO$_2$, on the other hand, is obtained by running the arterial blood on the oxygen sensitive electrode in the arterial blood gas machine.

Pulse Oximetry

Pulse oximetry tells us that what percentage of the hemoglobin is saturated with oxygen - SO_2. When it is measured in the arterial blood it is called SaO2. The following four principles illustrate the mechanism of pulse oximetry and its shortcomings -

1. The pulse oximeters routinely used in the hospitals have three components

      I. A source emitting two wavelengths of light i.e. red and infrared.
      ii. A receiver receiving these lights after they have passed through a part of the human body e.g. finger or ear lobule.
      iii. A computer processing unit which processes the information received from the receiver

2. The hemoglobin in the circulation is commonly found either in the oxidized (oxyhemoglobin / Oxy Hb) or the reduced (deoxyhemoglobin / Deoxy Hb) state. Oxyhemoglobin absorbs red light and deoxyhemoglobin infrared light.

3. When a part of human body with blood flowing through it e.g. fingertip, is placed between the emitting source and the receiver, part of the light from the emitting source is absorbed by the oxyhemoglobin (red light) and by the deoxyhemoglobin (infrared light). The remaining light falls on the receiver.

4. The computer in the processing unit calculates the saturation as follows-

$$SaO_2 \text{ (or } SpO_2) = \frac{Oxy\ Hb}{Oxy\ Hb + Deoxy\ Hb} \times 100$$

Since the pulse oximeter tells about the oxygen saturation of the hemoglobin in the **peripheral** circulation, it is also called SpO_2.

Contd.................

Pulse Oximetry continued :

Remember that

1. The **saturation reported on the ABG report SaO$_2$ is a calculated value** calculated from the PaO$_2$.

The PaO$_2$, SaO$_2$ (calculated from the PaO$_2$) and the SpO$_2$ (as read by the pulse oximeter) may all remain normal despite severe hypoxia at the tissue level. This can happen under a few clinically important but relatively uncommon circumstances. e.g. when carboxyhemoglobin (COHb) is present or if cyanide poisoning is present. Carboxyhemoglobin is present in blood in smokers in low concentration but higher value are seen in carbon monoxide poisoning. It is bright red in color and absorbs red light. It is therefore read as oxyhemoglobin by the pulse oximeter. Thus despite significant poisoning the SpO$_2$ remains normal. The correct saturation of hemoglobin by the oxygen (Oxy Hb) in such cases can be determined by using oximeter that emits four wavelengths. Two additional wavelengths record the concentration of carboxyhemoglobin (COHb) and methemoglobin (HbM or meth Hb). Thus the computer of the oximeter now reads as follows -

$$SpO_2 = \frac{OxyHb}{Oxy\ Hb + Deoxy\ Hb + COHb + Meth\ Hb} \times 100$$

Example : A patient with severe carbon monoxide poisoning has 8 gm% Oxy Hb, 2 gm% deoxy Hb, 4 gm% COHb. An ordinary pulse oximeter emitting light of two wavelengths will read a saturation of 80% . This is derived as follows-

$$\frac{8}{8+2} \times 100 = \frac{8}{10} \times 100 = 80\%$$

However, a pulse oximeter emitting light with four wavelengths will read the correct saturation which is 57%.

$$SpO_2 = \frac{8}{8+2+4} \times 100 = \frac{8}{14} \times 100 = 57\%$$

Contd.........

Pulse Oximetry continued :

MethHb is present in blood in excess either as a congenital disorder or in nitrate poisoning. It is blue in color and is read more like a deoxyHb and thus interferes with the correct reading by the pulse oximeter,

However, since these conditions are not very common in day to day practice, the pulse oximeter in routine clinical use emit lights of only two wavelengths i.e. red and infrared for oxyHb and deoxyHb, respectively.

2. Note, that since deoxygenated blood in venous circulation can cause problems in reading the saturation of the hemoglobin in the ARTERIAL circulation (SaO_2), the pulse oximeters are calibrated only to read the pulsatile wave form (arteries have pulsation but veins do not). This eliminates the interference arising from the venous circulation in reading SpO_2. However, the same principle makes it difficult to get a proper reading of SpO_2 from patients who have poor peripheral arterial circulation because of shock. Conversely, in patients with prominent venous pulsation as in those with severe tricuspid regurgitation or in those on positive pressure breathing with high inflation pressure, it may be difficult to get a correct SpO_2 reading from pulse oximeter.

3. Since the pulse oximeter reads only during the wave form or pulsation, the reading is not effected by static phenomenon like the amount of pigment in the skin or thickness of the finger or the ear lobule. The effect of nail polish is more related to the type and color of nail polish and varies from none to significant. In an emergency if you think that the nail polish is interfering with the reading of SpO_2 put the probe on the finger from side to side or put it on the ear lobule.

4. Pulse oximetry is quite reliable if the saturation of the hemoglobin is above 70 percent. Since such low SpO_2 are not permitted to last for long **(SpO_2 below 70% indicate severe hypoxia and must be corrected immediately by using whatever means that may be necessary including nasal cannula, ventimask or even by intubating the patient)** the inability of the pulse oximeters to read accurately below 70 % is not a big problem in a clinical setting.

Chapter 3 : Hemoglobin Oxygen Dissociation Curve

Normal Hemoglobin Oxygen Dissociation Curve
(Hb-O_2 dissociation curve)

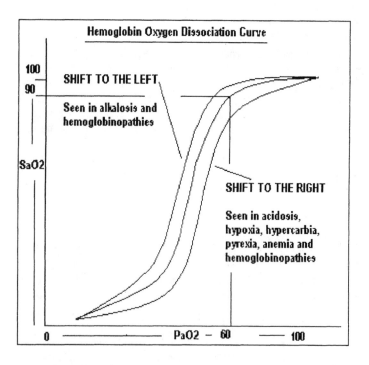

Dissociation between PaO$_2$ and SaO$_2$ could be because of either shift of the Hb - O$_2$ dissociation curve, because of the abnormally saturated hemoglobin or because of error in the measurement of PaO$_2$ and SaO$_2$ (see below).

Causes of Shift of Hemoglobin Oxygen Dissociation Curve:

Shift to the RIGHT : When the curve is shifted to the right the blood is able to release more oxygen in the tissues. Therefore, <u>in all conditions where tissue hypoxia is present, it will be the RIGHT thing for the curve to shift to the RIGHT</u>. These conditions include :

1. High altitude causes chronic hypoxia due to low absolute partial pressure of the oxygen in the air secondary to low atmospheric pressure. This causes an increase in 2,3 DPG concentration in the red cells. This rise in 2,3 DPG causes a change in the spatial configuration of the hemoglobin molecule which can now release more oxygen at the tissue level, thus helping the body fight the hypoxia. Similar mechanism applies in cases of chronic anemias also. (2,3 DPG = 2,3 Diphosphoglycerate).

2. Anemia - Tissue hypoxia due to low oxygen content of the blood i.e. decreased CaO_2.
(see later : $CaO_2 = 1.34 \times Hb$ in gm% $\times O_2$ sat/100 $+0.003 \times PaCO_2$)

3. Hypercarbia
4. Acidosis
5. Pyrexia
6. Abnormal hemoglobins (congenital)

Shift to the Left : Alkalosis is the commonest cause of shift of the curve to the left. Abnormal hemoglobin as in certain congenital hemoglobinopathies, methemoglobinemia and hereditary erythrocytosis are other important causes to remember.

Errors in the measurement of SaO_2 on the ABG : Although the error may be because of the instrument malfunction, clinically important conditions like the presence of abnormal hemoglobin e.g.. methemoglobin may also be responsible. Conversely, apparently normal results may be obtained in the presence of gross tissue hypoxia e. g. in the presence of carboxyhemoglobin or in cases of cyanide poisoning (see chapter on pulse oximetry)

Chapter 4 : HCO_3 and BE

<u>HCO_3 & BE</u> : Serum bicarbonate and Base Excess

These are calculated values from the pH and $PaCO_2$ by the Henderson-Hasselbach Equations :

$$pH = Constant\ K \times \frac{log\ HCO_3}{log\ H_2CO_3}$$

Thus, the HCO_3 on the ABG is the expected HCO_3 for that given pH and $PaCO_2$. In other words if the two values are given, the third one can be derived. That is what is done by the ABG machine while calculating the value of the HCO_3 from the pH and the $PaCO_2$.

Serum HCO_3 on the SMA6 is a more accurate measure of the ACTUAL HCO_3 as it is directly measured. Usually HCO_3 on the ABG is slightly lower than the HCO_3 on the SMA6. One explanation is that the bicarbonate estimation on SMA6 also includes estimation of the dissolved CO_2 in the plasma (in addition to the direct measurement of the actual bicarbonate in the serum).

$$CO_2 + H_2O === H_2CO_3 ==== H^+ + HCO_3$$

BASE EXCESS :

Similarly base excess is a calculated value and is not used very often for routine blood gas interpretation. This may be used to evaluate total body base excess or base deficit.

Chapter 5 : PaO_2

PaO_2 : Partial pressure of oxygen : Also, called PO_2. (For how to calculate it, see chapter on A -a DO_2).

One very important point to remember is that PaO_2 is the **partial pressure of oxygen in the PLASMA AND NOT IN THE WHOLE BLOOD**. Although this pressure determines the saturation of the hemoglobin in most circumstances they are **NOT INTERCHANGEABLE**. PaO_2 is the measure of dissolved oxygen in the plasma and is dependent on the pressure (P) at which the air is being inhaled and on the fraction of oxygen in the inspired air, FiO_2. This fact is used in the treatment of patients with carbon monoxide (CO) poisoning where due to the presence of carboxyhemoglobin, the tissue are unable to get oxygen (see chapter 9 on carbon monoxide poisoning). In these cases, high concentration of oxygen is used without (mild cases) or with (severe cases) high atmospheric pressures to increase the amount of oxygen dissolved in plasma (PaO_2). This dissolved oxygen is then delivered to the tissue (see chapter on relation of PaO_2, SaO_2 and CaO_2). Thus, inability of the hemoglobin to carry oxygen is bypassed by increasing the amount of O_2 dissolved.

Putting it as a picture in very simple terms :

Plasma carries dissolved oxygen i.e. $PaO2$.

MEASURED BY ARTERIAL BLOOD GAS ANALYSIS

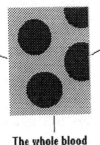

Red cells have hemoglobin which changes color depending on the saturation by the Oxygen i.e. $SaO2$.

MEASURED BY THE PULSE OXYMETRY

The whole blood

Once this fundamental is clear we can go ahead and ask " If PaO_2 supplies only about 0.3 ml of oxygen out of upto 5 ml needed by the tissue (see chapter 9 on O_2 content of the blood) then why do we measure it and rely on it for managing the patients?". The answer is simple - In most cases the PaO_2 corresponds with the hemoglobin saturation (in accordance to the Hb-O_2 dissociation curve) and therefore once we are aware of the pitfalls of the PaO_2 value we can use it. As mentioned in chapter one **'ALL BLOOD GAS VALUES MUST BE READ IN CONTEXT OF THE PATIENT'**. Again a patient may be severely hypoxic at the tissue level and die despite a normal PaO_2 value e.g. cyanide poisoning or carbon monoxide poisoning. Thus, the point about clinical correlation can not be overemphasized.

The significance of PaO_2 is that it indicates hypoxia and since the tissues, especially the brain, cannot tolerate hypoxia for long without sustaining a permanent damage, a low PaO_2 must always be corrected immediately. Depending on the severity of the hypoxia, the fraction of the oxygen in the inspired air (FiO_2) should be raised by nasal prongs / ventimask or nonrebreather mask. The patient may even be intubated to achieve a satisfactory PaO_2. Whatever means is used, the bottom line is that a PaO_2 of at least 60 or more should be maintained to prevent hypoxia associated injury to the tissue especially the brain.

Remember, that patients with tendency to retain carbon dioxide have respiratory center response to hypercarbia blunted and therefore they breathe because of their hypoxic drive. If this hypoxic drive is suddenly removed as by the rapid correction of the hypoxia then respiratory depression and even respiratory arrest can occur. In these patients one must start with lower oxygen concentration and increase or decrease the fractional inspired oxygen (FiO_2) gradually depending on the response of the PaO_2 and $PaCO_2$.

Beware of the following clinical situations while interpreting PaO_2:

A. If the blood sample is a venous sample then the PaO_2 will be around 40 and $PaCO_2$ around 45 with the blood pH around 7.35. However, an identical value may be obtained on blood gas analysis if the tissue hypoxia is severe. **Remember, the best way to decide whether the given sample is arterial or venous is to know that the sample has flown freely and passively into the syringe** and at no time the piston was withdrawn actively. Rarely, even this criteria does not hold true!

B. If there is an air-bubble in the syringe in which the blood is drawn for the ABG, the result of the PaO_2 will be higher than the true PaO_2 of the blood (PO_2 in the air bubble is equivalent to the atmospheric pressure x FiO_2 = 760 - 47 x 0.21 = 150 where 47 is the water vapor pressure).

C. If there is a high number of WBCs in the blood and the blood is made to stand for sometime before the ABG study is done, then the PaO_2 value will be lower than the true PaO_2 as the oxygen in the plasma will be consumed by those excessive WBCs to run their metabolic machinery.

D. Maximum possible PaO_2 while breathing "Room Air" is 150. Here is how it is derived :

| Partial pressure of a gas | = | Atmospheric pressure | x | Fraction of that gas in the atmosphere |

Oxygen forms 21 percent of the air we breathe. Thus, the FO_2 in air is 0.21.

| Partial pressure of oxygen in inspired air | = | Atmospheric pressure (Dry) | x | FiO_2 |

At the sea level the atmospheric pressure is 760 and the water vapor pressure is 47. Therefore, the atmospheric pressure of the dry air is 713.

Thus, PAO_2 = (760 - 47) x 0.21 = 713 x 0.21 = 150

Therefore, even if there is no hindrance to oxygen transfer across the alveolo-capillary membrane the maximum obtainable PaO_2 can not exceed 150 while breathing "Room Air" at the sea level (where water vapor pressure is 47). Here, it is presumed that there is no ventilation perfusion mismatch. In real life there is always some ventilation perfusion mismatch under normal circumstances (see dead space ventilation). Because of this fact the PaO_2 attained while breathing room air is always below 150 (when we breathe normally it is around 100 and is increased when someone hyperventilates as during a prolonged painful attempt of arterial puncture. However, as mentioned above it always remains below 150).

Thus, if any PaO_2 is reported as more than 150 then it was not drawn with the patient breathing room air and some effect of higher concentration of FiO_2 (common scenario) or higher atmospheric pressure (extremely rare in real practice but very important to understand the calculation of PAO_2 and A -a DO_2 A - a gradient).

Some Important Situations :

Theoretically speaking, if the patient is breathing 'Dry" air with no water vapor the maximally attainable PaO_2 at the atmospheric pressure will be 760 x 0.21 = 159.6. If this dry air is being inhaled at two atmospheric pressures e.g. in hyperbaric chamber, the maximally attainable PAO_2 will be 319 (2 x 760 x 0.21 = 319).

Similarly, if someone is breathing 100% O_2 e.g. a ventilated patient, without any humidification and there is (theoretically) no ventilation perfusion mismatch and no humidification of the inhaled gas in the patient's airways; then the maximal attainable PaO_2 will be (760 - 0) x 1.0 = 760. Again, in real life because of the humidification of the inspired air, dead space ventilation, perfusion of non aerated alveoli and the hindrance provided by the alveolo-capillary membrane such PaO_2 values are not achieved.

With the above concept it is easy to understand that why there is relative hypoxiemia at higher altitude where the atmospheric pressure is low. For example : at a height where the atmospheric pressure is half normal i.e. 760/2 = 380, the maximally attainable PiO_2 (Partial pressure of the inspired oxygen will be 380 x 0.21 = 79.8. As a result the maximally attainable PaO_2 will be less than 79.8 as the PaO_2 can not exceed PiO_2.

Since, the PiO_2 keeps decreasing as we go higher and higher, mountain climbers need supplemental oxygen and aircraft need to be pressurized.

EXERCISE : Calculate the maximal possible PaO_2 at a height where the atmospheric pressure is 75% of normal and the patient is breathing dry air.

ANSWER : Maximum possible PaO_2 = Maximal possible PAO_2
At 75% atmospheric pressure partial pressure of oxygen will be

(760 x 75/100 - 0) x 0.21 = 120

Here, other variables like water vapor pressure, $PaCO_2$, dead space ventilation, V/Q mismatch etc. are considered to be 0.

Chapter 6 : $PaCO_2$ and $PaCO_2$

PaCO$_2$: Partial pressure of carbon dioxide :

This simply indicates the patient's ventilation in relation to the CO_2 produced by the body. Since, under most circumstances the CO_2 production remains constant, $PaCO_2$ simply reflects the patient's ventilation.

Normal act of breathing includes -

i) Respiratory cycle is initiated in the respiratory center of the reticular activating system in the brain stem and then traverses in the spinal cord.

ii) The impulse to inhale travels in intercostal and phrenic nerves to neuromuscular junctions where membrane depolarization leads to muscular contraction of intercostal muscles and the diaphragm.

iii) As a result of muscular contraction during inspiration the diaphragm moves down (increasing the size of the chest cavity vertically) and contraction of the intercostal muscles make the ribs more horizontal (increasing the antero-posterior diameter of the chest).

Any condition which interferes with the above mechanism leads to hypoventilation which manifests as a rise in $PaCO_2$ on the blood gas analysis. **$PaCO_2$ is increased in conditions where the respiratory movements do not result into good flow of air into and out of the lungs - Hypoventilation.** This causes type II respiratory failure. An easy way to remember associated ABG abnormalities is that **type II respiratory failure has two types of abnormalities -**

1) Hypoxia (low PaO_2)
2) Hypercarbia (high $PaCO_2$)

Compare this with **type I respiratory failure which has only one abnormality** - Hypoxia (Low PaO_2).

Contd.....

Causes of hypoventilation or high $PaCO_2$:

i) Hypoventilation may be due to a weak central respiratory drive secondary to sedative or narcotic drug overdose (any central nervous depressant) or due to a head injury, raised intracranial pressure or cerebrovascular accident. It may also be due to blunting of the respiratory center's sensitivity to increased $PaCO_2$ as is seen in patients with chronic obstructive pulmonary disease.

Normally, a rise in the $PaCO_2$ should stimulate respiration to wash off this extra CO_2. This increased respiratory activity is mediated through the respiratory centers in the brain stem. In cases of COPD a rise in $PaCO_2$ fails to stimulate the respiration. In these patients the respiratory drive is maintained by the hypoxia and if this hypoxia is suddenly corrected the drive to breathe is lost and respiratory failure is precipitated. To avoid this **patients with COPD should be given oxygen very carefully and in lower concentration with a constant watch on their breathing pattern, PaO_2 and $PaCO_2$.**

ii) Hypoventilation could also be because the impulse generated in the brain stem can not reach the muscles of breathing -

- as in cervical cord injury
- radiculopathy-a common clinical example is Guillain-Barre` syndrome
- nerve problem as in bilateral phrenic nerve paralysis
- lower motor neuron involvement as in cases of late stages of motor neuron disease
- neuromuscular junction disorder as in myasthenia gravis
- muscle disease as in late myopathies
- fatigue of the respiratory muscles as in late stages of asthma can also lead to alveolar hypoventilation and an increase in $PaCO_2$.

iii) Despite intact neuromuscular pathways the thoracic cage may be so deformed that effective air flow in and out of the lungs can not occur. This occurs in severe kyphoscoliosis in the thoracic area. A relatively fixed chest wall as can occur in advanced ankylosing spondylitis can also cause hypoventilation and a rise in the $PaCO_2$.

Similarly a thick eschar of a chest burn, encasing the chest wall will lead to hypoventilation by physically limiting the expansion of the chest. Hypoventilation thus induced can be cured by escarotomy - splitting the scar surgically.

Causes of hyperventilation :

$PaCO_2$ is decreased in conditions associated with hyperventilation and is seen in the following clinical situations -

- anxiety disorder
- painful blood collection
- pulmonary embolism
- early stages of an attack of asthma
- early pneumonia
- ventilator malfunction
- pregnant females

In pulmonary embolism, pneumonia and asthma the hyperventilation may be secondary to the stimulation of receptors in the lung or may be due to mild hypoxiemia associated with these conditions. This hyperventilation tends to correct the hypoxemia and therefore these conditions may or may not show a decrease in PaO_2 (they usually do). On the other hand hyperventilation associated with anxiety is associated with either normal or a mild increase in the PaO_2.

Remember, in cases of pure acidosis a high $PaCO_2$ indicates hypoventilation in relation to CO_2 produced in the body, even though the patient may appear to be breathing normally.

As mentioned earlier the $PaCO_2$ tells about total ventilation in relation to the CO_2 produced. Thus, a patient may have high $PaCO_2$ and therefore hypoventilation, despite a respiratory rate of say thirty. This can occur if the ventilatory effort is not strong enough or for any other reason the air can not be moved in and out of the lungs. On the other extreme a relatively smaller patient may be hyperventilating even if ventilating at the rate of say ten if the ventilator tidal volume is set too high for him. Thus, it is important to understand and remember that **respiratory rate alone does not tell us about hypo or hyper ventilation in terms of the carbon dioxide produced in the body and therefore the $PaCO_2$.**

Chapter 7 : The pH

pH is defined as negative logarithm of the hydrogen ion concentration. We will come back to this concept later in this chapter. pH tells about the acidity or alkalinity of a medium.

Normal pH varies from 7.35 to 7.45. Death is imminint at pH of below 6.9 or above 7.9. It must be remembered that the pH, like any other component of the ABG must be read in the clinical context. For example - a patient may have a pH of 7.2 secondary to a chronic respiratory problem without the need for artificial ventilation; the same pH if occurs because of acute respiratory failure may need immediate artificial ventilation. Similarly, in the post-ictal state (post-seizure) the pH of the arterial blood may be quite low e.g. 7.0 but usually does not need intubation or ventilation as it is rapidly corrected on its own once the seizure is over and normal respiratory activity is established. Thus, although there is no magic number below or above which any certain type of therapy is indicated in all cases, definitive therapy is indicated at a pH below 7.15 or above 7.6. Again, it is the overall clinical picture which decides the next best step for the management of the patient.

pH as mentioned above is negative logarithm of the hydrogen ion concentration. Thus, a small change in the pH indicates a significant change in the hydrogen ion concentration. Thus, a pH change from 7.4 to 7.1 indicates doubling of the hydrogen ion concentration from 40 to 80 mmol/l.

Acidosis is the process which either adds acid or removes alkali from the body fluids. This leads to a state of plasma called 'Acidemia'. Alkalosis is the reverse of that. Thus, alkalosis is the process that either adds alkali or removes acid from the body fluids and thus results into 'Alkalemia'. For practical purposes we have used the terms acidosis and alkalosis (rather than acidemia and alkelemia) as they are the terms used commonly in a day to day practice.

The concept of hydrogen ion concentration rather than the pH is gaining more and more importance and is therefore explained here in detail. One advantage of knowing the H^+ concentration is that the validity of the ABG can be checked (see below).

pH v /s hydrogen ion concentration (H⁺) :

An easy formula to remember the relationship between the pH and the Hydrogen ion concentration is -

Change in pH by 0.1 = Change in hydrogen ion concentration by 20%

For example :   pH H^+ concentration

pH	H^+ concentration
7.0	**100**
7.1	80
7.2	64
7.3	50
7.4	**40**
7.5	30
7.6	24
7.7	20

Thus, a pH decrease of 0.1 causes the hydrogen ion concentration to increase by 20% and an increase of the pH by 0.1 causes them to decrease by 20%. Note that in the above table 20, 24, 30, 40, 50, 64, 80 and 100 are 20 percent higher or lower from the value before or after them.

According to Henderson-Hasselbalch equation :

$$H^+ ion\ conc = constant\ K \times \frac{PaCO_2}{HCO_3}$$ (Constant K has a fixed value of 24)

PaCO2 of	HCO_3 of	H^+ will be	Calculation for H^+ will be	Approximate pH (See table above)
40	24	40	24x40/24=40	7.4
60	24	60	24x60/24=60	7.2
20	24	20	24x20/24=20	7.7
40	16	60	24x40/16=60	7.2
60	16	90	24x60/16=90	7.05
20	16	30	24x20/16=30	7.5

If the $PaCO_2$, HCO_3, H^+ do not have the above relationship the blood gas report is not correct and should be repeated. This is an easy way to check the validity of the given blood gas report.

Chapter 8 : Alveolo- arterial oxygen gradient : A-a DO$_2$

A-aDo$_2$ is also called A-a gradient.

Theoretically speaking if there was no barrier to the transport of oxygen from the alveolus to the blood, the maximum PaO$_2$ that could be attained breathing room air will be 150 as that is the partial pressure of oxygen in the inspired air (PiO$_2$).

$$
PiO_2 = \begin{array}{c} \text{Atmospheric pressure} \\ \text{in mm of Hg} \\ \text{(Normal value 760)} \end{array} - \begin{array}{c} \text{water vapor} \\ \text{pressure} \\ \text{at sea level} \\ \text{(Normal 47)} \end{array} \times \begin{array}{c} FiO_2 \\ \text{(Normal 0.21)} \end{array}
$$

$PiO_2 = (760 - 47) \times 0.21 = 713 \times 0.21 = 150$

However, in real life PaO$_2$ of 150 cannot be achieved as the following factors play a role :

i) Alveolar membrane offers some resistance to the transfer of the oxygen from the alveolar space to the blood. This becomes important in conditions where this membrane is damaged or is thickened e.g. pulmonary fibrosis or pulmonary edema.

ii) There is some CO$_2$ in the blood which prevents free transfer of the oxygen. Thus the formula is not PAO$_2$ = PaO$_2$ but it is as follows :

A-aDo$_2$ = PAO$_2$ - PaO$_2$ - 1.25 PaCO$_2$

Note that 1.25 PaCO$_2$ can be written as PaCO$_2$ + 0.25 PaCO$_2$
or still simpler form will be 1.25 PaCO$_2$ = PaCO$_2$ + $\dfrac{PaCO_2}{4}$

Thus   **A-aDO$_2$ = PAO$_2$ - PaO$_2$ - PaCO$_2$ - $\dfrac{PaCO_2}{4}$**

If you remember this formula you can calculate the alveolo arterial oxygen gradient (A-aDO$_2$) without using a pen or a calculator. That's how I do it ! In all exams, including the boards, help from calculators and graphs is prohibited. **This also applies to the graph for the reading of the ABGs!**

Example : ABG on room air : pH 7.40 / $PaCO_2$ 40/ PaO_2 90
A-a DO_2 = 150 - 90 -40 -40/4 = 150 -90-40-10 = 10

3. Ideally all the alveolar units that have blood supply should be ventilated and all the alveoli that are ventilated should be perfused. Under certain physiological (upper lung alveoli are aerated more and lower lung alveoli are perfused more) and pathological conditions (either the alveolar space is obliterated or the supplying vessel is blocked) a ventilation perfusion mismatch occurs.

The alveolus is filled with pus in pneumonia, fluid in pulmonary edema, blood in pulmonary hemorrhage, inflammatory exudate in pneumocystis pneumonia but is still being perfused normally as the blood supply to the alveolus is not effected; this unit of lung will have perfusion but no ventilation and the A-aDO_2 will increase. On the other hand there may be a patient with pulmonary embolism, the embolus causing non- perfusion of the normally aerated alveolus leading to ventilation but no perfusion. This **mismatch between ventilation and perfusion is CLINICALLY THE MOST IMPORTANT CAUSE OF ABNORMALLY HIGH A-a GRADIENT.**

Importance of calculating the A -a gradient is clear from the fact that a normal A -a gradient means that the lungs are normal and the cause for the problem lies somewhere else. Conversely, an abnormal A -a gradient indicates a problem in the lungs. Take for example a patient who has a very high $PaCO_2$ but the A- a gradient is normal. Immediately look for a problem outside the lung. Conversely, a patient where you are suspecting say narcotic overdose leading to coma - a high A - a gradient should immediately make you think of associated lung problem e. g. aspiration.

However, if any condition causes equal loss of lung parenchyma and the vasculature the A -a gradient may remain normal as there is no ventilation perfusion mismatch.

The normal value for the A-a gradient varies with age but normally is 10 to 20 mm of Hg. One easy formula to remember is -

$$A - a DO_2 = \frac{Age}{4} + 4$$

Thus, if a patient is 40 years old the normal A-aDO_2 is upto 10 but if he is 80 years old the normal value goes up to 24 and in a 100 year old upto 29.

Thus to conclude :

$$A - a\ DO_2 = \text{Atmospheric pressure} - \text{Water Vapor Pressure} \times FiO_2 - PaO_2 - 1.25\ PaCO_2$$

$$= (760 - 47) \times 0.21 - PaO_2 - PaCO_2 - \frac{PaCO_2}{4}$$

$$= 713 \times 0.21 - PaO_2 - PaCO_2 - \frac{PaCO_2}{4}$$

$$\mathbf{= 150 - PaO_2 - PaCO_2 - \frac{PaCO_2}{4}}$$

Although, the most important cause of abnormal A - a DO_2 is pulmonary embolism, many lung pathologies including pneumonia, pulmonary embolism, pulmonary edema, pulmonary hemorrhage and many more can cause an abnormal A - a gradient.

Now calculate theoretical A -a gradient in a patient breathing dry room air (no water vapor) at two atmosphere pressures. His PaO_2 is 200 and $PaCO_2$ is 40.

Answer :

$$A -a\ DO_2 = (P_B - WVP) \times FiO_2 - PaO_2 - PaCO_2 - \frac{PaCO_2}{4}$$

$$= (760 \times 2 - 0) \times 0.21 - 200 - 40 - 40/4$$

$$= (760 \times 2) \times 0.21 - 200 - 40 - 10$$

$$= 1520 \times 0.21 - 250 = 319.2 - 250 = 69.2$$

Chapter 9 : Relation Between PaO_2, SaO_2 and CaO_2

PaO_2 = partial pressure of oxygen in the blood plasma
SaO_2 = saturation of the hemoglobin in the blood
CaO_2 = oxygen content of the blood

As mentioned earlier PaO_2 is the partial pressure of the oxygen in the plasma and is estimated directly by the ABG machine by running the blood on the oxygen sensitive electrode. In other words when we say that PaO_2 is 90 we mean that the oxygen is putting a partial pressure of 90 mm of Hg in that patient's plasma.

Depending on the position of SaO_2 in relation to the PaO_2 on the hemoglobin - Oxygen dissociation curve this pressure PaO_2 determines that to how much extent the hemoglobin gets saturated / oxidized by the oxygen i.e. SaO_2. The SaO_2 is either obtained by the pulse oximeter or is derived by the simple mathematical calculation from the PaO_2 and reported on the arterial blood gas report. Both these methods have shortcomings which should be appreciated (See chapter on PaO_2 and pulse oximetry).

CaO_2 on the other hand is the total amount of oxygen carried by the blood and is calculated by the following formula :

$$CaO_2 = (Hb \times 1.34 \times SaO_2) + 0.003 \times PaO_2$$

Considering a Hb of 14 and SaO_2 of 99 as in a normal person the oxygen carried by the hemoglobin will be 14 x 1.34 x 0.99 = 18.57 ml.

Compare this with the oxygen carried dissolved in the plasma. This will be 0.003 x 100 (normal PaO_2 is 100 approximately) = 0.03 ml only. Thus, a major portion of oxygen to be supplied to the tissues is carried with the hemoglobin. However, under certain circumstances the oxygen carried in the plasma can be increased several fold and this property is used in the treatment of carbon monoxide poisoning (see below).

Contd........

Carbon monoxide poisoning, Hyperbaric Oxygen therapy and Oxygen content of the blood :

Carbon monoxide is generated when a carbon containing substance burns in the absence of sufficient oxygen. In the blood the carbon monoxide (CO) combines with the hemoglobin forming carboxyhemoglobin (COHb). The binding of the carbon monoxide to the hemoglobin is almost two hundred times stronger than oxygen. This binding also shifts the hemoglobin oxygen dissociation curve to the left thereby decreasing oxygen release at the cellular level. This is in addition to the hypoxia caused due to a loss of binding site for oxygen on the hemoglobin molecule. Both these lead to hypoxia at the cellular level resulting into anaerobic metabolism and lactic acidosis.

Although, minimal elevation in carbon monoxide in the blood occur in smokers, toxic exposure occurs when coal, petroleum or wood (all rich in carbon) is burnt in an environment lacking enough oxygen. This is an important poisoning; especially in the elderly in the winter season. Deaths have occurred by exposure in small garages when the car engine is left running in the absence of ventilation or even when carbon monoxide has leaked into the passenger compartment of the car from the exhaust system.

One important clue to the poisoning comes from history of headache and symptoms of cold starting in many family members SIMULTANEOUSLY.

If carbon monoxide poisoning is suspected routine pulse oximetry should not be used to monitor the patient as it will give falsely high readings for the SaO_2 (see chapter on pulse oximetry).

Carbon monoxide poisoning can be mild, moderate or severe. Whereas the milder forms can be treated with inhalation of high flow oxygen by the face mask (e.g.. 10 l/mt), more severe forms (with neurologic symptoms including altered mental status and / or cardiovascular changes like ischemia or arrhythmias or patients with high carbon monoxide levels should be treated with intubation and ventilation with 100 percent oxygen.

In severe carbon monoxide poisoning, hyperbaric oxygen therapy (oxygen at higher atmospheric pressures e.g. 2 or 3) should be used. This has two advantages. It accelerates the process of dissociation (CO from Hb) which would have taken many hours now gets completed in a few minutes. Equally important is the fact that that much more oxygen is now carried in the plasma and thus the tissue hypoxia is prevented. We have seen earlier (chapter 9, oxygen content of the blood) that at one atmospheric pressure plasma carries 0.3 ml of oxygen /dl (O_2 carried in plasma = PaO_2 x 0.003 = 100 x 0.003 = 0.3)

However, if the patient breaths dry 100 percent oxygen at a pressure of two atmosphers then theoretically maximum possible PaO_2 will be 1520. That is, PiO_2 = (760 x 2 - 0) x FiO_2 = 1520 x 1.0 = 1520. If we presume all this PiO_2 can be transferred to the blood the blood PaO_2 will be 1520. At that PaO_2 the blood will be able to carry 1520 x 0.003 = 4.56 ml of oxygen.

For the sake of simplicity in the above examples water vapor pressure, dead space ventilation, $PaCO_2$ are considered as 0.

Remember, always to speak of FiO_2 (fraction of oxygen in inspired air) in terms of fraction of 1 and NOT AS PERCENTAGE. Thus FiO_2 in a patient on a hundred percent oxygen is 1.0 and NOT 100. Also, a patient breathing room air has an FiO_2 of 0.21 and NOT 21 percent. A patient on 50 percent ventimask has an FiO_2 of 0.5 and not 50 percent.

Chapter 10 : Basics of Reading an ABG Report

Normal parameters on an ABG report are -

Parameter	Normal range	Mean
pH	7.35 - 7.45	7.40
$PaCO_2$	35 - 45	40
HCO_3	22-28	25

Some consider the normal range for the pH to be 7.38 to 7.42 and the normal range for $PaCO_2$ to be 38 to 42. However, all changes in the pH, $PaCO_2$ and HCO_3 should be calculated from the mean.

How to read the ABGs :

Rule 1 : Look at the pH
   1A - If the pH is less than 7.35 there is acidosis.
   1B - If the pH is more than 7.45 there is alkalosis
   1C - If the pH is 7.35 to 7.45 there is a :
                  C1 - either a combined acid base disorder
                  C2 - there is no acid base disorder
                  C3 - there is complete compensation for the acid base disorder

Rule 2 : Look at the $PaCO_2$
   2A - If the $PaCO_2$ is increased with acidosis there is respiratory acidosis
   2B - If the $PaCO_2$ is decreased with a decreased pH there is metabolic acidosis
   2C - If the $PaCO_2$ is decreased with alkalosis there is respiratory alkalosis
   2D - If the $PaCO_2$ is increased with alkalosis there is metabolic alkalosis
   2E - If the $PaCO_2$ is 35 -45 with a normal pH there is probably no acid base disorder (see below) or there are two disorders moving the $PaCO_2$ in the opposite directions e.g. metabolic acidosis and metabolic alkalosis or respiratory acidosis and respiratory alkalosis

Rule 3 : Look at the change in the pH for 10 mm change in PaCO$_2$

In acute respiratory failure, carbon dioxide accumulates. This forms carbonic acid and leads to acidosis. If the problem causing retention of CO_2 persists the body adjusts by forming and retaining HCO_3 , mainly in the kidneys. This causes the pH to return **towards** normal. Thus, for a given rise in PaCO$_2$, the fall in blood pH is reduced. This is obvious below in rule 3A and 3B. Rule 3A shows that if the **pH falls by 0.07 for 10 mm rise in PaCO$_2$, it is acute respiratory acidosis**. Over time this fall in the pH is corrected by a rise in HCO_3. Thus, in chronic respiratory acidosis, for a 10 mm rise in PaCO$_2$ the pH falls by 0.03 only (Rule 3B). Any fall in the pH between 0.03 and 0.07 for 10 mm rise in PaCO$_2$ will be due either to a partially compensated respiratory acidosis or due to acute on chronic (mixed) respiratory acidosis.

Change in pH for 10 mm change in PaCO$_2$

| | RESPIRATORY | | METABOLIC |
	Acute	Chronic	Acute or Chronic
Acidosis	0.07 (Rule 3A)	0.03 (Rule 3B)	The two digits of the pH after the decimal are the same as the PaCO$_2$. (Rule 3E)
Alkalosis	0.08 (Rule 3C)	0.03 (Rule 3 D)	Same as above 3E (Rule 3 F)

Rule 4 : Look for change in HCO$_3$ for 10 mm change in PaCO$_2$

| | RESPIRATORY | | METABOLIC | |
	Acute	Chronic	Acute	Chronic
Acidosis	1-1.2 (Rule 4A)	3 - 4 (Rule 4B)	10 (Rule 4C)	10 (Rule 4D)
Alkalosis	2.5 (Rule 4E)	5.0 (Rule 4F)	14 (Rule 4G)	14 (Rule 4H)

Contd.......

The change in bicarbonate for a given changes in pH or $PaCO_2$ tells whether there is compensation or not; and if there is compensation, whether it is appropriate and complete or not. If the compensation is not appropriate then a mixed disorder should be looked for.

The above can be summarized as follows :

pH	Acidosis/ alkalosis	$PaCO_2$	HCO_3	Disorder
Decreased	Acidosis	Increased	Increased	Respiratory acidosis
Decreased	Acidosis	Decreased	Decreased	Metabolic acidosis
Increased	Alkalosis	Increased	Increased	Metabolic alkalosis
Increased	Alkalosis	Decreased	Decreased	Respiratory alkalosis

To simplify it further :

Since it is obvious from the above table that $PaCO_2$ and HCO_3 move in the same direction, the above can be summarized as follows -

$PaCO_2$ or HCO_3	Decreased pH (Acidosis)	Increased pH (Alkalosis)
Decreased	Metabolic	Respiratory
Increased	Respiratory	Metabolic

LIMITS OF COMPENSATION :

- During respiratory acidosis, CO_2 is retained. This causes an increase in HCO_3. During acute respiratory acidosis, the HCO cannot rise above 30. However, during the chronic phase of the acidosis the kidneys retain HCO_3 and it can rise up to 55.

- During respiratory alkalosis, the $PaCO_2$ falls due to hyperventilation. However, it cannot fall below 16 to 18 mm of Hg. Lower $PaCO_2$ cause increase in pH. At higher pH tetany may occur due to a fall in fraction of ionised calcium.

- During metabolic acidosis, deep and frequent breathing occurs, causing a fall in the $PaCO_2$. However, the $PaCO_2$ does not fall below 10 - 12 in adults and about 6 - 8 in children

- During metabolic alkalosis, hypoventilation occurs causing an increase in $PaCO_2$. The $PaCO_2$ cannot rise above 55, as further hypoventilation is prevented by hypoxia.

- Values of HCO_3 and $PaCO_2$ beyond those described can be seen in mixed acid base disorders.

- When a disorder compensates, **there is never an overcompensation**. In other words if patient tries to correct for respiratory acidosis by retaining bicarbonate, then he will never retain so much bicarbonate as to cause alkalosis.

How to approach an acid base disorder :

1. Look at the pH
2. Look at the $PaCO_2$
3. Look at the HCO_3
4. Evaluate degree of compensation or correction
5. Evaluate the ABG for a mixed acid base disorder

For a stepwise approach to the ABG please see the next page.

How to approach an acid base disorder on the ABG

```
Look at the pH
!
!--- Below 7.35 ---there is acidosis
!     !
!     look at the PCO2
!         !
!         !---Above 45 means acidosis is respiratory
!         !           !
!         !           Look for increase in HCO3 for
!         !           10 mm increase in PCO2 to evaluate
!         !                 -if 1-1.2 --Acute resp acidosis
!         !                 -if 1.3-3 --Partial compensation
!         !                 -if 3.1-4.0 --Full compensation
!         !
!         !---Below 35 means acidosis is metabolic
!         !      In pure metabolic acidosis
!         Rule i)PCO2 is the same as two digits of
!                the pH after the decimal
!         Rule j)or PCO2 = (1.5xHCO3)+8+2
!         Rule k)or PCO2=HCO3+15 if HCO3 is above 10
!
!---Above 7.45 means that there is alkalosis
!     !
!     Look at the PCO2
!         !
!         !---Below 35 means alkalosis is respiratory
!         !     !
!         !     !--look for fall in HCO3 for 10 mm
!         !     !  fall in PCO2
!         !     !      -if 2.5--- acute resp alkalosis
!         !     !      -if 5--- chronic resp alkalosis
!         !     !
!         !     !--Look for rise in pH for 10 mm fall
!         !            of PCO2
!         !                 -if 0.08--Acute resp alkalosis
!         !                 -if 0.03--Chronic resp alkalosis
!         !
!         !---Above 45 means alkalosis is metabolic
!                Expected PCO2 = 0.7x HCO3+20+1.5
!
!---7.35 to 7.45 - possibilities can be
                    a)No acid base disorder
                    b)Compensated disorder
                    c)Mixed disorder
                (See exercise 9, 10 and 11 below)
```

Section II

Blood Gas Interpretation Made Easy

Chapter 11 : Respiratory Acidosis

Ex 1 : ABG   pH 7.28 $PaCO_2$ 60   HCO3 27

Step	Observation	Interpretation
1.	pH is below 7.35	There is acidosis (Rule 1A)
2.	$PaCO_2$ is increased	Acidosis is respiratory (Rule 2A)
3.	$PaCO_2$ is increased by 20 from 40 and the HCO_3 by 2 from 25. Thus the HCO_3 rise by 1 for 10 mm rise in $PaCO_2$	The compensation is full (Rule 4A) for acute respiratory acidosis. The HCO_3 did not have enough time to rise. Therefore, the marked fall in the pH.
4.	pH has fallen by 0.12 from 7.4 for 20 mm rise in $PaCO_2$ from a mean of 40 (0.06 for a 10 mm rise in $PaCO_2$)	This is appropriate compensation for acute respiratory acidosis (Rule 3A)

Diagnosis : Pure acute respiratory acidosis

Causes of respiratory acidosis are causes of hypoventilation (see chapter 6 on $PaCO_2$). Note that during **acute** respiratory acidosis, for the pH to fall from 7.40 to 7.28 the PaCO2 has increased from 40 to 60. For a similar fall in the pH during **chronic** respiratory acidosis, the $PaCO_2$ rises upto 80 (see exercise 2 on the next page). This is due to a rise in the HCO_3 from 27 to 39 from acute to chronic respiratory acidosis. This process takes a few days and helps the pH to return towards normal.

Ex 2 : ABG   pH 7.28   PaCO$_2$ 84   HCO$_3$ 39

Step	Observation	Interpretation
1.	pH is below 7.35	There is acidosis (Rule 1A)
2.	PaCO$_2$ is increased	Acidosis is respiratory (Rule 2A)
3.	PaCO$_2$ is increased by 44 from 40 and HCO$_3$ by 14 from 25. Thus the rise in HCO$_3$ is 3.2 for 10 mm rise in PaCO$_2$	The compensation is full (Rule 4B) for chronic respiratory acidosis. The HCO$_3$ has risen well so the effect on the pH is much lesser despite a very high PaCO$_2$ of 84.
4.	pH has fallen by 0.12 (from mean 7.4) for 44 mm (from 40) rise of PaCO$_2$ i.e 0.028 for 10 mm change in PaCO$_2$	Change in pH is appropriate for it to be chronic respiratory acidosis (Rule 3B)

Diagnosis : Pure chronic respiratory acidosis.

Causes of respiratory acidosis : These are basically the causes of hypoventilation (see chapter 6 on PaCO$_2$). Note here that the HCO3 has risen from 25 to 39 and as a result the effect on the pH has been much lesser despite a much higher PaCO2 (compare ABG reports in exercise 1 and 2 above).

Chapter 12 : Metabolic Acidosis

Ex 3 : ABG   pH 7.30 $PaCO_2$ 30   HCO3 15

Step	Observation	Interpretation
1.	The pH is below 7.35	There is acidosis (Rule 1A)
2.	$PaCO_2$ is decreased	Acidosis is metabolic (Rule 2B)
3.	I) $PaCO_2$ value is the same as the last two digits after the decimal in the pH (Rule 3E)	The numbers are correct for it to be pure metabolic acidosis according to rule 3E.
	ii) HCO_3 + 15 = $PaCO_2$ Here HCO_3 is 15 and $PaCO_2$ is 30.	15 + 15 = 30. Rule K (see algorithm) is satisfied.
	iii) $PaCO_2$ = 1.5 HCO_3 + 8 Here, 1.5 x HCO_3 + 8 is 22.8 + 8 or 30.5(Rule J)	Measured $PaCO_2$ is 30 and calculated 30.5. Rule J is satisfied. Therefore it is pure metabolic acidosis.

Diagnosis : Pure metabolic acidosis

Remember that **as soon as you diagnose metabolic acidosis you must calculate the anion gap.** This will immediately classify the acidosis into two classes -

1. Anion gap metabolic acidosis or **AGMA**
2. Non anion gap metabolic acidosis or **NAGMA**

Contd........

The concept of anion gap :

It must be clear from the very beginning that **no such gap really exists in the body** (In - vivo) and this is only a concept - an **In-Vitro phenomenon** (In- vitro = outside the body).

Normally, there are positively and negatively charged ions in our body. Positively charged ions are called **CATIONS and include Sodium, Potassium, Calcium, Magnesium, globulins** and many more including minerals and rare elements.

Negatively charged ions are called **ANIONS and include Chloride, Bicarbonate, Sulfate, Phosphate, Albumin** and other organic ions which are produced in the body as a result of metabolism.

Total number of anions in the body equals the total number of cations and if each and every anion and cation is accounted for, there will be no anion gap. This, however would be very cumbersome, time consuming and financially impractical. Therefore, we only estimate the major cations and anions for calculating the anion gap. We subtract the major anions (Chloride and HCO_3 110 and 25 meq respectively) from major cations (sodium 140 meq) and label the difference as anion gap. Thus, this **gap represents those negatively charged ions (anions) in the body which are balancing the electric charge of the positively charged ions (cations) but are not estimated** (see picture on the next page).

Thus **Anion gap = Na - Cl - HCO_3**

Normal anion gap is 12 ± 4 i.e. 8 to 16. Some consider the normal range to be 10 to 14.

In cases with **pure anion gap metabolic acidosis, the rise in anion gap from 12 should equal the fall in HCO_3 from 24.** If there is significant discrepancy then a mixed disorder should be considered. **This is the principle behind the concept of gap-gap which is expressed as a ratio of change in anion gap to the change in HCO_3 .**

In pure anion gap metabolic acidosis this ratio remains as one. Considering that in a patient the anion gap is 30, the change in serum bicarbonate will make the ratio above or below one (for details see the book 'Understanding Water and Electrolytes Made Easy' by the same author). **Thus the gap-gap helps us decide about the mixed acid base disorders**.

Anion Gap

TOTAL CATIONS (in body) = TOTAL ANIONS

Other cations like globulins, K etc* not used in calculation of anion gap		Other anions like Albumin, SO4, PO4 etc* not used in the calculation of anion gap
	Anion gap 16	
		HCO3=24
Na=140		Cl=100

Contd.....

Causes of increased anion gap :

The anions may be added to the body and therefore to the blood, from an outside source (exogenous) or from within the body as a result of metabolism (endogenous). Although, there is a common neumonic to remember the causes as **MUDPILES** (Methanol, Uremia, Diabetic ketoacidosis, Paraldehyse, Iron or INH, Lactic acidosis, Salicylates), it is much more important to understand the pathophysilogy of the process. The above neumonic puts less important and less common causes first. Further, more important causes are not distinguished. Also, one alphabet represents more than one important clinical disorder e.g. 'S' stands for salicylates, sepsis and starvation. A much better neumonic, which is clinically oriented, will be - **DARLINGS ARE IMP (ortant)**.

D	Diabetic keto acidosis
A	Alcohol
R	Renal failure
L	Lactic acidosis from any cause
I	Iron poisoning
N	No food (starvation)
G	Generalized seizures
S	Sepsis
A	Aspirin poisoning
R	Rhabdomyolysis
E	Ethylene glycol
I	INH
M	Methanol
P	Paraldehyde

Important endogenous sources of anions include:

Cause	Anion accumulated
1. Cardiopulmonary failure	- Lactate
2. Renal failure	- Organic acids, SO_4, PO_4
3. Diabetes Mellitus	- Keto acids
4. Starvation	- Keto acids
5. Anaerobic metabolism	- Lactate

Important exogenous sources of anions include :

Cause	Anion accumulated
1. Salicylates	- Salicylic acid
2. Ethanol	- Keto and lactic acid
3. Methanol	- Formic acid
4. Ethylene glycol	- Glycolic and oxalic acid
5. Paraldehyde	

All the above are causes of AGMA (anion gap metabolic acidosis). **In all cases of high anion gap, look for measured serum osmolality and its difference from calculated serum osmolality. The difference is called the osmolal gap and it is increased if the blood have substances with osmolality different from that of plasma and if these substances are not used in calculationg serum osmolality, e.g. ethanol** which has osmolality of 23 or methanol with osmolality of 34 mOsm (approximately) at 100 mg/dl blood level.

$$\text{Serum Osmolality (Calculated)} = 2 \times Na + \frac{Glucose}{18} + \frac{Urea}{2.8}$$

Contd....

Measuring serum osmolality directly additionally measures osmolality imparted by other osmotically active substances such as alcohols. Therefore, **measured serum osmolality is higher than calculated serum osmolality if the patient has consumed alcohol.** The degree of increse in osmolality varies and depends on the type of alcohol in the blood. Each 100 mg% of ethanol increase osmolality by23. Corresponding rise in osmolality by methanol and isopropyl alcohol are 34 and 18 (approximately).

$$\text{Serum Osmolality} = 2\times Na + \frac{Glucose}{18} + \frac{Urea}{2.8} + \text{other osmotically}$$
$$\text{(Measured)} \qquad\qquad\qquad\qquad\qquad \text{Active substances}$$

Remember that **salicylates give an anion gap metabolic acidosis but do not increase osmolality**. On the other hand **Isopropyl alcohols increase serum osmolality but do not increase the anion gap**. Ethanol and methanol increase both the osmolality and the anion gap.

Isopropyl alcohol is the common rubbing alcohol on hospital wards. Methanol is used as a de-icing agent in windshield fluids and ethylene glycol is used as antifreeze in cars.

Albumin is a negatively charged particle (anion). In the serum it counterbalances the cations (e.g. Na) but is not used as a component of negatively charged ions while calculating the total number of anions.Therefore, it is responsible (along with some other anions) for the anion gap phenomenon. As a result **when serum albumin significantly decreases the anion gap decreases too**. Converesely, globulins are positively charged particles (cation) and their increase (globulins) causes a decrease in the anion gap. **Sometimes, a low anion gap is the first clue to the presence of increased globulins or paraproteins (e.g. multiple myeloma) in the body**. Always remember, as said earlier, if we measure all the cations and anions in the serum there will be no anion gap as all the cations will balance all the anions.

Non Anion Gap Acidosis : NAGMA :

In the conditions causing NAGMA there is **acidosis, but** the balance between sodium on one side and chloride and bicarbonate on the other is not disturbed. The loss of bicarbonate is compensated by a rise in chloride. Therefore, the **anion gap (Na - Cl - HCO_3) is not changed.** Important causes of loss of bicarbonate include :

1. Gastrointestinal losses
    - Diarrhea
    - Small bowel fistula
    - Continuous small bowel drainage
    - Ileostomy
    - Uretrosigmoidostomy
    - Ileal conduit for ureter

2. Urinary losses
    - Proximal renal tubular acidosis
    - Distal renal tubular acidosis
    - Acetozolamide therapy
    - Urinary obstruction

Sometimes, both an anion gap acidosis and non-anion-gap acidosis are present together in the same patient e.g. Diabetic ketoacidosis in a patient with renal tubular acidosis. The clue to the disorder comes from the fact that the **fall in HCO_3 is excessive for the given degree of anion gap** (both from the mean) when other causes of low HCO_3 e.g. respiratory alkalosis have been excluded. For example, if a patient has an anion gap of 18 (6 above a mean of 12) then the expected HCO_3 will be 19 (6 below mean of 25). If, however, the patient's serum HCO_3 is 12 and there is only pure metabolic acidosis; then consider the presence of both anion gap and non anion gap metabolic acidosis.

Chapter 13 : Respiratory Alkalosis

Ex 4 : ABG   pH 7.54   PaCO$_2$ 25   HCO$_3$ 21

Step	Observation	Interpretation
1.	The pH is above 7.45	There is alkalosis (Rule 1B)
2.	PaCO$_2$ is decreased	Alkalosis is respiratory (2C)
3.	PaCO$_2$ is decreased by 15 from 40 and the HCO$_3$ by 4 from 25. Thus the fall in HCO$_3$ is 2.7 for 10 mm fall in PaCO$_2$	The compensation is full (Rule 4E) for acute respiratory alkalosis. The HCO$_3$ did not have enough time to fall therefore the marked rise in the pH.
4.	For a 15 mm fall in PaCO$_2$ the pH has gone up by 0.14 from 7.4 i.e. a rise of pH of 0.09 for 10 mm fall in PaCO$_2$	There is appropriate compensation for pure acute respiratory alkalosis (Rule 3C)

Diagnosis : Pure acute respiratory alkalosis.

Causes of respiratory alkalosis can either be nonpulmonary or pulmonary. Non pulmonary causes include hysteric hyperventilation or CNS disorders like encephalitis. Pulmonary causes include pulmonary embolism, early pneumonia and early stages of bronchial asthma. Remember, **a pH that is normal or towards respiratory acidosis in a patient with a severe attack of asthma is a dangerous sign and indicates impending respiratory failure with a possible need for intubation and ventilation.** Similarly, **if in an asthmatic the initial low PaCO$_2$ on ABG is normalizng and the patient's clinical condition is getting worse than probably respiratory exhaustion is setting in causing hypoventilation and increasing the PaCO$_2$.**

Ex 5 : ABG   pH 7.46   PaCO$_2$ 20   HCO$_3$ 15

Step	Observation	Interpretation
1.	The pH is above 7.45	There is alkalosis
2.	PaCO$_2$ is decreased	Alkalosis is respiratory
3.	PaCO$_2$ is decreased by 20 from 40 and HCO$_3$ by 10 from 25. Thus, the fall in HCO$_3$ is 5 for 10 mm fall in PaCO$_2$	The compensation is full (Rule 4F) for chronic respiratory alkalosis. The HCO$_3$ has fallen enough; therefore, the minimal rise in the pH. Compare this with exercise 4 above.
4.	For a 20 mm fall in PaCO$_2$ the pH has gone up by 0.06 from 7.4 i.e. rise in pH of 0.03 for 10 mm fall in PaCO$_2$	There is appropiate compensation for pure chronic respiratory alkalosis (Rule 3D).

Diagnosis :Pure chronic respiratory alkalosis.

In respiratory alkalosis the compensation becomes complete in about two weeks and the pH returns **towards** normal.

The lowest PaCO$_2$ achieved by hyperventilating is approximately 16.

Chapter 14 : Metabolic Alkalosis

Ex 6 : ABG   pH 7.56   PaCO$_2$ 55   HCO$_3$ 45

Step	Observation	Interpretation
1.	pH is above 7.45	There is alkalosis (Rule 1B)
2.	PaCO$_2$ is increased	Alkalosis is metabolic (Rule 2C)
3.	PaCO$_2$ value is the same as the last two digits of the pH after the decimal point	The compensation is full (Rule 3F) for pure metabolic alkalosis
4.	PaCO$_2$ is increased by 15 from 40 and HCO$_3$ by 20 from 25. Thus the rise in HCO$_3$ is 14 for 10 mm rise in PaCO$_2$	The compensation is full (Rule 4G/H) for metabolic alkalosis

Diagnosis : Pure metabolic alkalosis

Whenever you diagnose metabolic alkalosis look for urinary chloride to decide whether the alkalosis will respond to administration of chloride or not. **The commonest cause of metabolic alkalosis in clinical practice is diuretic therapy.** They respond well to the stopping of the diuretic. Another very common cause is volume contraction due to dehydration.

Causes of Metabolic Alkalosis :

Common causes of metabolic alkalosis can be divided into chloride responsive and chloride resistant depending on whether the urine chloride is below or above 15 meq/l.

Chloride responsive metabolic alkalosis is associated with low urinary chloride (below 15 meq/l) and include :

- vomiting
- continuous nasogastric suction
- volume contraction states

Chloride resistant metabolic alkalosis is associated with urinary chloride above 15 meq/l and occurs in :

- hypercortisolism
- hyperaldosteronism
- sodium bicarbonate therapy
- severe renal artery stenosis

Exception : The case with metabolic alkalosis with use of diuretics is a special one. Since they are natriuretic, diuretics increase urinary loss of sodium and chloride. However, the alkalosis induced by them responds to administration of saline. Thus, **despite a high urinary chloride the alkalosis responds to chloride administration**.

Chapter 15 : Mixed Acid Base Disorders

Ex 7 : ABG   pH 7.2 $PaCO_2$ 80 HCO_3 32

Step	Observation	Interpretation
1.	pH is below 7.35	There is acidosis
2.	$PaCO_2$ is increased	Acidosis is respiratory
3.	$PaCO_2$ is increased by 40 from 40 and the HCO_3 has increased by 7 from 25. Thus the rise in HCO_3 is 1.8 for 10 mm rise in $PaCO_2$	For acute respiratory acidosis HCO_3 should rise by 1 and for chronic respiratory acidosis by 3 to 4 for a 10 mm rise in $PaCO_2$ (Rule 4A,4B). A rise of 1.8 could either be due to a partial correction of an acute respiratory acidosis by compensation or may be due to acute-on-chronic respiratory acidosis.
4.	$PaCO_2$ rise of 40 is matched with a pH fall of 0.2 from 7.4 i.e. a fall in pH of 0.05 for 10 mm rise in $PaCO_2$	In acute respiratory acidosis for 10 mm rise in $PaCO_2$ the pH falls by 0.07 and in chronic phase by 0.03. Fall of 0.05 may either be due to an acute-on-chronic respiratory failure or due to incomplete (Rule 3A, 3B) compensation

Diagnosis :   *Acute -on-chronic respiratory acidosis*
Or
Partially compensated acute respiratory acidosis

Ex 8 : ABG   pH 7.2 $PaCO_2$ 50 HCO_3 19

Step	Observation	Interpretation
1.	pH is below 7.35	There is acidosis
2.	$PaCO_2$ is increased	Acidosis is respiratory
3.	$PaCO_2$ is increased by 10 from 40 but HCO_3 is decreased. In simple disorders $PaCO_2$ and HCO_3 always move in the same direction i.e. either increased or decreased	If the disorder is pure respiratory acidosis the HCO_3 with this rise in $PaCO_2$ of ten should be 26-30 (Rule 4A/4B) but it is only 19. Thus a mixed disorder is present. On top of respiratory acidosis there is a disorder decreasing the HCO_3. It could either be metabolic acidosis or respiratory alkalosis (either of them can decrease the HCO_3)
4.	$PaCO_2$ rise of 10 is matched with pH fall of 0.2 from 7.4. If it is pure respiratory acidosis maximum fall in pH possible is 0.07. Here, the fall in pH is much more	The fall in the pH is out of proportion to expected due to respiratory acidosis. Therefore, an additional disorder causing acidosis is present which is associated with a fall in HCO_3. Metabolic acidosis fits all these criteria.

Diagnosis : *Mixed disorder with respiratory acidosis and metabolic acidosis*

Ex 9 : ABG   pH 7.45 $PaCO_2$ 70 HCO_3 50

Step	Observation	Interpretation
1.	pH is normal at 7.45	3 possibilities can be a) No acid base disorder b) Compensated disorder c) Mixed disorder
2.	$PaCO_2$ is increased	Possibility (a) is excluded. There is an acid base disorder (b) or(c).
3.	$PaCO_2$ is increased by 30 (70 from 40) and HCO_3 by 25 (50 from 25). Thus, for 10 mm rise in $PaCO_2$ the HCO_3 has insreased by 8.	If it is compensated respiratory acidosis, the HCO_3 value with this rise in $PaCO_2$ of 30 can at the most be 37 (Rule 4B) but it is 50. Thus, a mixed disorder is present. On top of respiratory acidosis there is a disorder increasing the HCO_3 and increasing the pH from acidosis to alkalotic side. Metabolic alkalosis fits all these criteria
4.	$PaCO_2$ rise of 30 is associated with pH rise of 0.05 from 7.4. If there is pure resp acidosis possible fall in the pH could be from 0.1 to 0.21. Here the pH has rather risen by 0.05	The change in the pH is in the opposite direction of expected due to respiratory acidosis. Therefore, an additional disorder causing alkalosis is present which is associated with a rise in HCO_3. Metabolic alkalosis fits all these criteria.

Diagnosis : *Mixed disorder with respiratory acidosis and metabolic alkalosis.*

Chapter 16 : Miscellaneous Disorders

Ex 10 : ABG   pH 7.35 $PaCO_2$ 50 HCO_3 28

Step	Observation	Interpretation
1.	pH is normal at 7.35	3 possibilities can be a) No acid base disorder b) Compensated disorder c) Mixed disorder
2.	$PaCO_2$ is increased	Possibility (a) is excluded. There is an acid base disorder (b) or (c).
3.	$PaCO_2$ is increased by 10 from 40 and HCO_3 by 3 from 25	If it is compensated respiratory acidosis, then with a 10 mm rise in $PaCO_2$ the HCO_3 can be 26 to 29 (acute to chronic disorder - Rule 4A, 4B). Here it is 28. Thus it is compensated respiratory acidosis.
4.	$PaCO_2$ rise of 10 is associated with pH fall of 0.05 from 7.4	The fall in the pH is as expected ie 0.03 to 0.07 (Rule 3A, 3B) for respiratory acidosis. There is no mismatch. Therefore this is fully compensated respiratory acidosis.

Diagnosis : Compensated respiratory acidosis

Ex 11 : ABG   pH 7.38 $PaCO_2$ 39 HCO_3 23

Step	Observation	Interpretation
1.	pH is normal at 7.38	4 possibilities are a) No acid base disorder b) Compensated disorder c) Mixed disorder d) Wrong ABG report
2. 3.	$PaCO_2$ is normal HCO_3 is normal	Probably there is no acid base disorder (Rule 2E). Also, see below.
4.	H^+ for a pH of 7.38 will be 42. (See chapter 7 on pH and H^+ concentration - pH of 7.3 and 7.4 correspond to a H+ of 50 and 40 respectively).	$H^+ = \dfrac{24 \times PaCO_2}{HCO_3}$ OR $H^+ = \dfrac{24 \times 39}{23} = 41$ (See chapter 7 on pH and H^+ concentration)

Diagnosis : No evidence of an acid base disorder on the ABG analysis.

Correlate clinically. Rare possibility of metabolic acidosis (which will decrease the pH, $PaCO_2$ and HCO3) and metabolic alkalosis (which will increase the pH, $PaCO_2$ and HCO_3) occuring together cannot be excluded. .

Ex 12 : ABG   pH 7.6 $PaCO_2$ 35 HCO_3 32

Step	Observation	Interpretation
1.	pH is 7.6	There is alkalosis
2.	$PaCO_2$ is decreased 5 mm from a mean of 40	There is respiratory alkalosis (next - look for compensation).
3.	$PaCO_2$ is decreased by 5 from 40 and HCO_3 is increased by 7 from 25	If it is compensated respiratory alkalosis, HCO_3 should fall by 1.2 to 2.5 with 5 mm fall in $PaCO_2$ (Rule 4E, 4F). However, here it has rather risen by 7. Thus a mixed disorder is present. On top of resp alkalosis there is a disorder increasing the HCO_3. The other disorder that can cause such a change is metabolic alkalosis
4.	$PaCO_2$ fall of 5 is associated with a pH rise of 0.2 from 7.4. If it was pure resp alkalosis the rise in pH should have been 0.015 to 0.04 (Rule 3C, 3D). However, here the pH has risen by 0.2	The rise in the pH is much more than expected. Therefore an additional disorder causing a rise in the pH and rise in HCO_3 (see point 3 above) is present. Metabolic alkalosis fits all these criteria.

Diagnosis : Mixed disorder with respiratory alkalosis and metabolic alkalosis.

Ex 13 : ABG from a healthy 24 year old female
pH 7.4 $PaCO_2$ 28 HCO_3 16

Step	Observation	Interpretation
1.	pH is 7.4	Normal pH
2.	$PaCO_2$ is decreased	3 possibilities can be a) Metabolic acidosis with respiratory alkalosis b) very early stage of hyperventilation c) wrong ABG report
3.	HCO_3 is decreased	Since it takes time to decrease the HCO_3 the second possibility is ruled out. Also note that the pH is normal.
4.	The patient is healthy	First possibility is unlikely.
5.	Is the ABG report correct? $H^+ = \dfrac{24 \times PaCO_2}{HCO_3}$ should hold true (see chapter on pH)	Here H^+ ion concentration is ~40 (corresponds to a pH of 7.4) $H^+ = \dfrac{24 \times 28}{16} = 42$ The relationship hold true. Thus ABG report is correct.
6.	Go back to the clinical picture. She is a young healthy female	Could it be that she is pregnant? In pregnany the $PaCO_2$ decreases. This is probably due to the effect of progestrone. The pH is maintained normal by a corresponding fall in the HCO_3.

Diagnosis : Normal ABG in a pregnant female

Ex 14 : ABG   pH 7.5   PaCO$_2$ 20   HCO$_3$ 22

Step	Observation	Interpretation
1.	pH is 7.5	The patient has alkalosis
2.	PaCO$_2$ is decreased	Patient has respiratory alkalosis
3.	For 10 mm fall in PaCO$_2$ the pH rises by 0.08 in acute and 0.03 in chronic (3C, 3D) respiratory alkalosis.	Looks like partially compensated respiratory alkalosis as for 20 mm fall in PaCO$_2$ the pH has gone up by 0.1 from 7.4 or the rise in pH is 0.05 for 10 mm change in PaCO$_2$.
4.	HCO$_3$ has fallen by 1.5 for a PaCO$_2$ fall of 10	If it is pure respiratory alkalosis the HCO$_3$ should have fallen by 2.5 to 5 for a 10 mm fall in PaCO$_2$ (4E, 4F).
5.	Is this ABG reading correct?	pH of 7.5 corresponds to H$^+$ of 30 (see chapter 7 on the pH). In this case calculated H$^+$ = 24xPaCO$_2$/ HCO$_3$ i.e. 24x20/22 = 21.8 only. Therefore, this ABG report is not correct.

Diagnosis : Wrong ABG report.

If the report is not fully evaluated and only the pH and the PaCO$_2$ are taken into consideration, then the report would have been passed as a partially compensated respiratory alkalosis. If the PaCO$_2$ and HCO$_3$ readings are correct than the pH would be 7.68 or so and if the pH and HCO$_3$ are correct the PaCO$_2$ should have been 32 (all calculated by the formula H$^+$= 24 x PaCO$_2$/HCO$_3$)

Notes

Section III

Exercises

Exercise A

Now attempt to solve the following exercises on your own without the help from the book. On the next page are the answers and explanations.

Ex 1 : ABG   pH 7.28 PCO_2 60 HCO_3 27

Ex 2 : ABG   pH 7.28 PCO_2 84 HCO_3 39

Ex 3 : ABG   pH 7.3 PCO_2 30 HCO_3 15

Ex 4 : ABG   pH 7.54 PCO_2 25 HCO_3 21

Ex 5 : ABG   pH 7.46 PCO_2 20 HCO_3 15

Ex 6 : ABG   pH 7.56 PCO_2 55 HCO_3 45

Ex 7 : ABG   pH 7.2 PCO_2 80 HCO_3 32

Ex 8 : ABG   pH 7.2 PCO_2 50 HCO_3 19

Ex 9 : ABG   pH 7.45 PCO_2 70 HCO_3 50

Ex 10 : ABG   pH 7.35 PCO_2 50 HCO_3 28

Ex 11 : ABG   pH 7.38 PCO_2 39 HCO_3 24

Ex 12 : ABG   pH 7.6 PCO_2 35 HCO_3 32

Ex 13 : ABG from a 24 year old healthy female
     pH 7.4 PCO_2 28 HCO_3 16

Ex 14 : ABG   pH 7.5 PCO_2 20 HCO_3 22

Answers to exercise A

Ex 1 : ABG   pH 7.28 PCO_2 60 HCO_3 27
Diagnosis : Pure acute respiratory acidosis.

Ex 2 : ABG   pH 7.28 PCO_2 84 HCO_3 39
Diagnosis : Pure chronic respiratory acidosis.

Ex 3 : ABG   pH 7.3 PCO_2 30 HCO_3 15
Diagnosis : Pure metabolic acidosis.

Ex 4 : ABG   pH 7.54 PCO_2 25 HCO_3 21
Diagnosis : Pure acute respiratory alkalosis.

Ex 5 : ABG   pH 7.46 PCO_2 20 HCO_3 15
Diagnosis : Pure chronic respiratory alkalosis.

Ex 6 : ABG   pH 7.56 PCO_2 55 HCO_3 45
Diagnosis : Pure metabolic alkalosis.

Ex 7 : ABG   pH 7.2 PCO_2 80 HCO_3 32
Diagnosis : Acute -on-chronic respiratory acidosis
                              Or
Partially compensated acute respiratory acidosis.

Ex 8 : ABG   pH 7.2 PCO_2 50 HCO_3 19
Diagnosis : Mixed disorder with respiratory acidosis and
                metabolic acidosis.

Answers to exercise A continued

Ex 9 : ABG   pH 7.45 PCO_2 70 HCO_3 50
Diagnosis : Mixed disorder with respiratory acidosis and metabolic alkalosis.

Ex 10 : ABG   pH 7.35 PCO_2 50 HCO_3 28
Diagnosis : Compensated respiratory acidosis

Ex 11 : ABG   pH 7.38 PCO_2 39 HCO_3 24
Diagnosis : No evidence of an acid base disorder on the ABG analysis. Correlate clinically.

Ex 12 : ABG   pH 7.6 PCO_2 35 HCO_3 32
Diagnosis : Mixed disorder with respiratory alkalosis and metabolic alkalosis.

Ex 13 : ABG from a healthy 24 year old female
pH 7.4 PCO_2 28 HCO_3 16
Diagnosis : Normal ABG in a pregnant female

Ex 14 : ABG   pH 7.5 PCO_2 20 HCO_3 22
Diagnosis : Wrong ABG report.

If this report is not fully evaluated and only the pH and the $PaCO_2$ are taken into consideration, then the report would have been passed as a partially compensated respiratory alkalosis. If the PCO_2 and HCO_3 readings are correct than the pH should be 7.68 or so; and if the pH and HCO_3 are correct the PCO_2 should be 32. (all calculated by the formula $H^+ = 24 \times PaCO_2/HCO_3$)

For detailed explanations see the corresponding exercise numbers on the previous pages.

Exercise B

S No	pH	PCO$_2$	HCO$_3$	Acid base disorder is.....
1.	7.3	30	14	
2.	7.5	20	14	
3.	7.6	20	17	
4.	7.6	30	28	
5.	7.5	50	36	
6.	7.45	80	54	
7.	7.3	80	37	
8.	7.23	75	30	
9.	7.4	40	24	
10.	7.25	63	26	
11.	7.25	45	19	
12.	7.38	12	24	

Answers to Exercise B

S No	pH	PCO_2	HCO_3	Acid base disorder is.....
1.	7.3	30	14	Metabolic acidosis
2.	7.5	20	14	Chronic resp alkalosis
3.	7.6	20	17	Acute resp alkalosis
4.	7.6	30	28	Acute resp alkalosis and Metabolic alkalosis
5.	7.5	50	36	Metabolic alkalosis
6.	7.45	80	54	Metabolic alkalosis and Chronic resp acidosis
7.	7.3	80	37	Chronic resp acidosis
8.	7.23	75	30	Acute on chronic resp acidosis or partially compensated acute respiratory acidosis
9.	7.4	40	24	Normal ABG report. Correlate clinically
10.	7.25	63	26	Acute resp acidosis
11.	7.25	45	19	Resp and metabolic acidosis
12.	7.38	12	24	Wrong report. pH and HCO_3 are normal. PCO_2 can not be 12.

Exercise C

Identify possible acid base disorders in the following cases -

1. JD a 68 year old man with chronic obstructive pulmonary disease and chronic renal failure presented to the emergency room. An arterial blood gas reading on admission, breathing room air was as follows -
pH 7.22   PCO$_2$ 52   PaO$_2$ 50   HCO$_3$ 20   SaO$_2$ 82%

2. TM, a 36 year old AIDS patient admitted with an altered mental state. Room air ABGs were as follows -
pH 7.15   PCO$_2$ 36   PaO$_2$ 70   HCO$_3$ 12   SaO$_2$ 86%

3. DN, a 45 year old cirrhotic admitted with vomiting for three days and altered mental status. Room air blood gases were -
pH 7.56   PCO$_2$ 36   PaO$_2$ 98   HCO$_3$ 27   SaO$_2$ 96%

4. BN, a 25 year old female patient admitted with dyspnea for six hours. Room air ABGs showed -
pH 7.6   PCO$_2$ 30   PaO$_2$ 106   HCO$_3$ 28   SaO$_2$ 99%

5. HS, a 68 year old patient who has been a heavy smoker all his life presents with the following ABGs -
pH 7.36   PCO$_2$ 50   PaO$_2$ 78   HCO$_3$ 28   SaO$_2$ 88%

6. TE, a 62 year old with cor pulmonale came to the ER with complaints of cough and phlegm. Room air ABGs showed -
pH 7.24   PCO$_2$ 78   PaO$_2$ 68   HCO$_3$ 32   SaO$_2$ 80%

7. A patient with 'acute exacerbation of COPD' had to be intubated for respiratory failure. Immediate post intubation ABGs showed -
pH 7.15   PCO$_2$ 56   PaO$_2$ 268   HCO$_3$ 18   SaO$_2$ 99.9%

Exercise C continued

8. HD, a 28 year old female being treated for anxiety disorder presented to the ER. An ABG was done as the oxygen saturation was low. The report was -
pH 7.58 PCO_2 22 PaO_2 54 HCO_3 20 SaO_2 70%

9. TG, a 44 year old asthmatic patient who continues to smoke four cigarettes a day was admitted for surgical removal of an ovarian mass. The ABG showed -
pH 7.44 PCO_2 22 PaO_2 58 HCO_3 14 SaO_2 72 %

10. MN, a 68 year old patient came to the ER on a cold December morning complaining of headache every morning. His wife living with him has similar symptoms for the same duration. An ABG showed -
pH 7.44 PCO_2 37 PaO_2 86 HCO_3 23 SaO_2 97 % (calculated).
What will you do next?

Answers to exercise C

1. Mixed disorder - Respiratory and metabolic acidosis.

2. Mixed disorder - Metabolic and respiratory acidosis.

3. Mixed disorder - Respiratory and metabolic alkalosis.

4. Mixed disorder - Respiratory and metabolic alkalosis.

5. Compensated chronic respiratory acidosis.

6. Partially compensated respiratory acidosis.

7. Mixed disorder - Metabolic and respiratory acidosis.

8. Acute respiratory alkalosis.

9. Chronic respiratory alkalosis

10. Probably carbon monoxide poisoning in an old person who has been trying to keep warm by heating his room with fire from coal or wood with inadequate ventilation in the room. We will immediately order measured SaO_2 and an estimation of carboxyhemoglobin.

Remember, **not to diagnose the ABG by clinical associations alone**. For example, a patient with AIDS can be short of breath with respiratory alkalosis not only because of a pneumocystis carinii (PCP) pneumonia but also because of hysteric hyperventilation, bronchial asthma or pulmonary embolism. He can have respiratory acidosis from a drug overdose or metabolic acidosis from septecemia.

Exercise D

---

1. PL, a 82 year old man with congestive heart failure was admitted with early pneumonia. Patient was on lasix, digoxin and coumadin. Admission ABG included -
pH 7.6 H^+ 24 PCO_2 35 PaO_2 56 HCO_3 32 SaO_2 70%

2. HY a 32 year old pregnant patient with hyperemesis presented with tingling in both hands . Room ait ABG showed -
pH 7.5 H^+ 30 PCO_2 50 PaO_2 96 HCO_3 37 SaO_2 98%

3. WT, a 27 year old asthmatic patient admitted to the hospital with shortness of breath. Admission ABGs were -
pH 7.4 H^+ 40 PCO_2 30 PaO_2 76 HCO_3 18 SaO_2 88 %

4. Patient WT in the above exercise no.3 continued to have low saturation on pulse oxymeter. ABG on 5 L/mt O_2 by nasal cannula now shows -
pH 7.4 H^+ 40 PCO_2 48 PaO_2 52 HCO_3 26 SaO_2 68 %

5. Patient WT in the above exercise placed on 50% ventimask with only minimal improvememt in saturation. The patient also appeared lethargic. ABG showed -
pH 7.28 H^+ 54 PCO_2 54 PaO_2 62 HCO_3 24 SaO_2 74 %

6. Above patient WT was intubated and put on 100 percent O_2 (FiO_2 = 1.0). The blood gas 14 hours later showed -
pH 7.5 H^+ 30 PCO_2 24 PaO_2 362 HCO_3 19 SaO_2 99.9 %

7. BE, a 28 year old female patient under treatment for anxiety disorder presented to the ER after an argument with her employer. She complained of spasms in both her hands. The ABG showed -
pH 7.52 H^+ 28 PCO_2 25 PaO_2 112 HCO_3 20 SaO_2 99.9 %

Contd ....

Exercise D continued

---

8. RI, a 78 year old patient with COPD, cor pulmonale came to the ER with history of shortness of breath and yellow phlegm. He was on digoxin and metalazone for the congestive heart failure and was waiting in the triage area for an hour. The ABG while breathing room air showed -
pH 7.32 H^+ 48 PCO_2 56 PaO_2 172 HCO_3 327 SaO_2 91%

9. SR, a 32 year old patient with history of recurrent admissions for drug overdoses came to the ER with altered mental status. ABG on room air showed -
pH 7.1   H+ 80 PCO_2 66 PaO_2 62 HCO_3 20 SaO_2 78 %

10. GT, a 86 year old person living alone found to be confused by the emergency medical services brought to the ER. Patient was discharged after the (PTCA) percutaneous transluminal coronary angioplasty three months ago. He now complains of severe chest pains which occur at rest and are relieved by sublingual nitrate tablets. He looks comfortable and is in no apparent distress.
pH 7.28 H^+ 54 PCO_2 58 PaO_2 62 HCO_3 26 SaO_2 78 %

Answers to Exercise D

---

1. Mixed metabolic and respiratory alkalosis with hypoxia.

2. Pure metabolic alkalosis.

3. Acute respiratory alkalosis.

4. Acute respiratory acidosis superimposed on respiratory alkalosis leading to a normal pH with raised PCO_2. This is dangerous sign in an asthmatic.

5. Acute respiratory acidosis in an asthmatic secondary to respiratory failure due to respiratory muscle fatigue. This patient may soon need respiratory support.

6. Acute respiratory alkalosis secondary to hyperventilation on the ventilator. If the patient's respiratory rate is high, the ventilator (in assist control mode) will be repeatedly triggered causing hyperventilation. (See book on ventilators by the same author).

7. Respiratory alkalosis due to hyperventilation.

8. Wrong report. The PaO_2 while breathing room air cannot be 172.

9. Mixed respiratory and metabolic acidosis.

10. Methemoglobinemia due to excess nitrate ingestion. There is also respiratory acidosis. Almost 50 % PTCA restenose in the first 6 months. This patient was using excessive nitrates to relieve his anginal pain. Respiratory acidosis is incidental.

Exercise E

Calculate the alveolo arterial oxygen gradient for the following patients who live at the sea port of Dover.

S No	pH	PCO_2	HCO_3	PaO_2	FiO_2	A-aDO_2
1.	7.3	30	14	80	Room Air	
2.	7.5	20	14	440	1.0	
3.	7.6	20	17	120	Room Air	
4.	7.6	30	28	200	0.4	
5.	7.5	50	36	130	0.3	
6.	7.45	80	54	100	0.4	
7.	7.3	80	37	70	0.4	
8.	7.23	75	30	80	0.5	
9.	7.4	40	24	90	0.3	
10.	7.25	63	26	320	0.6	

Answers to Exercise E

S No	pH	PCO_2	HCO_3	PaO_2	FiO_2	$AaDO_2$
1.	7.3	30	14	80 Air	Room	32
2.	7.5	20	14	440	1.0	248

1. $(760 - 47) \times 0.21 - 80 - 30 - 30/4 = 32$

2. $(760 - 47) \times 1.0 - 440 - 20 - 20/4 = 248$

Remember, that at very high FiO_2 values this formula does not apply very accurately. The purpose of this exercise is to make you understand the principle of calculating A - a gradient (A - a DO_2).

S No	pH	PCO_2	HCO_3	PaO_2	FiO_2	$AaDO_2$
3.	7.6	20	17	120 Air	Room	5
4.	7.6	30	28	200	0.4	48
5.	7.5	50	36	130	0.3	21
6.	7.45	80	54	100	0.4	85
7.	7.3	80	37	70	0.4	115
8.	7.23	75	30	80	0.5	183
9.	7.4	40	24	90	0.3	74
10.	7.25	63	26	320	0.6	29

4. $(760 - 47) \times 0.4 - 200 - 30 - 30/4 = 47$

5. $(760 - 47) \times 0.3 - 130 - 50 - 50/4 = 21$

Exercise F

Calculate the oxygen content of the whole blood (CaO$_2$) in the following cases -

S. No	pH	PCO$_2$	HCO$_3$	PaO$_2$	Hb gm %	Atmos pheric pressure	SaO$_2$	CaO2
1.	7.3	30	14	90	14	1.0	97	
2.	7.5	20	14	70	12	1.0	92	
3.	7.6	20	17	900	15	2.0	99	
4.	7.6	30	28	900	10	2.0	99	
5.	7.5	50	36	800	15	1.5	70	
6.	7.45	80	54	100	14	1.0	99	
7.	7.3	80	37	80	16	1.0	94	
8.	7.23	75	30	70	16	1.0	91	
9.	7.4	40	24	50	12	1.0	70	
10.	7.25	63	26	60	14	1.0	82	

Answers to Exercise F

S. No	pH	PCO_2	HCO_3	PaO_2	Hb gm %	Atmos pheric pressure	SaO_2	CaO_2
1.	7.3	30	14	90	14	1.0	97	18.4

$(14 \times 1.34 \times 0.97) + 0.003 \times 90 = 18.19 + 0.27 = 18.46$

2.	7.5	20	14	70	12	1.0	92	15.0

$(12 \times 1.34 \times 0.92) + .003 \times 70 = 14.79 + .21 = 15.0$

3.	7.6	20	17	900	15	2.0	99.9	22.7

$(15 \times 1.34 \times .0.999) + 0.003 \times 900 = 20.08 + 2.7 = 22.7$
Note the significant contribution made by the O_2 dissolved in the plasma ie 2.7 ml

4.	7.6	30	28	900	10	2.0	99.9	16.08

$(10 \times 1.34 \times 0.99) + 0.003 \times 900 = 13.38 + 2.7 = 13.38$

5.	7.5	50	36	800	15	1.5	70	16.47

$(15 \times 1.34 \times 0.7) + 0.003 \times 800 = 14.07 + 2.4 = 16.47$

Compare this with exercise F1 above. Note that low oxygen content carried by the hemoglobin (14.07 compared to 18.19) is counterbalanced by increasing the oxygen dissolved in the plasma (2.4 ml compared to 0.27 ml in exercise F1) by increasing the atmospheric pressure. If high FiO_2 is added, much more dissolved oxygen can be carried in the plama. This principle is used in the treatment of carbon monoxide poisoning.

Contd........

Answers to Exercise F continued

S. No	pH	PCO$_2$	HCO$_3$	PaO$_2$	Hb gm %	Atmos pheric pressure	SaO$_2$	CaO$_2$
6.	7.45	80	54	100	14	1.0	99	18.87
	$(14 \times 1.34 \times 0.99) + 0.003 \times 100 = 18.57 + 0.3 = 18.87$							
7.	7.3	80	37	80	16	1.0	94	20.3
	$(16 \times 1.34 \times 0.94) + 0.003 \times 80 = 20.1 + 0.24 = 20.3$							
8.	7.23	75	30	70	16	1.0	91	19.7
	$(16 \times 1.34 \times 0.91) + 0.003 \times 50 = 19.51 + 0.15 = 11.4$							
9.	7.4	40	24	50	12	1.0	70	11.4
	$(12 \times 1.34 \times 0.7) + 0.003 \times 50 = 11.25 + 0.15 = 11.4$							
10.	7.25	63	26	60	14	1.0	82	15.6
	$(14 \times 1.34 \times 0.82) + 0.003 \times 60 = 15.4 + 0.18 = 15.58$							

Exercise G

Compare the following clinical conditions (1 to 15) with the corresponding blood gas reports (a to n). Choose the **most appropriate** answer -

1. Salicylate poisoning
2. Cardiac arrest
3. Ventilator malfunction
4. Alcohol intoxication
5. Drug overdose, no loss of conciousness
6. Alcohol intake followed by blindness
7. Some alcohol intake followed by acute renal failure
8. Drug overdose with loss of consciousness
9. Bronchial asthma
10. Sepsis
11. Status epilepticus
12. Diarrhea
13. Diuretics
14. Addison's disease
15. Cushing's syndrome

a) Respiratory acidosis and metabolic acidosis
b) Respiratory alkalosis and metabolic acidosis with anion gap
c) Respiratory acidosis with no A-a gradient
d) Respiratory acidosis with A-a gradient
e) High anion gap metabolic acidosis with osmolal gap
f) High osmolal gap
g) Metabolic acidosis
h) Respiratory alkalosis or respiratory acidosis
I) Metabolic acidosis or metabolic alkalosis
j) Metabolic alkalosis, hypokalemia, high urine chloride
k) Metabolic acidosis and hypokalemia
l) Metabolic acidosis with hyperkalemia
m) Metabolic alkalosis, hypokalemia, low urine chloride
n) Respiratory acidosis, metabolic acidosis, myocardial infarction
o) Respiratory acidosis or alkalosis, low peak expiratory flow rate

Answers to exercise G

1.	Salicylate poisoning	B
2.	Cardiac arrest	N
3.	Ventilator malfunction	H
4.	Alcohol intoxication	E
5.	Opioid overdose, no loss of conciousness	C
6.	Alcohol intake followed by blindness	E
7.	Some alcohol intake followed by acute renal failure	F
8.	Opiod overdose with loss of conciousness	D
9.	Bronchial asthma	P
10.	Sepsis	G,I
11.	Status epilepticus	A
12.	Diarrhea	K
13.	Diuretics	J
14.	Addison's disease	L
15.	Cushing's syndrome	M

In the above example more than one answers can be correct. Emphasis is placed on the most appropriate answer. Cardiac arrest cause metabolic acidosis but it also leads to respiratory arrest. Similarly seizures cause metabolic acidosis but prolonged attack can be associated with respiratory failure (transient) with or without aspiration.

Space available here and the scope of this book does not permit a full discussion of the above disorders. For that refer to a text book of medicine. You may also refer to 'Fluids And Electrolytes Made Easy' by the same author.

Remember

While looking at the ABG always consider the clinical picture and determine the following -

1. Is the patient hypoxic?
2. What is the FiO_2 ?
3. Is the PaO_2 appropiate for the given FiO_2 ?
4. What is the alvelo arterial gradient?
5. What is the relation of the PaO_2 to SaO_2 and SpO_2?
6. Is the oxygen content of blood adequate to prevent hypoxia at the tissue level?
7. Is the patient hypoventilating / hyperventilating or ventilating normally for his $CO2$ production?

While analysing an acid base disorder determine the following -

1. The disorder is pure or mixed.
2. The disorder is respiratory or metabolic.
3. The disorder is acute or chronic, if respiratory.
4. If metabloic acidosis, what is the anion gap.
5. If metabolic alkalosis then is it chloride responsive i.e. what is the urine chloride.
6. Does the H+ ion concentration correspond to the PCO2 and the HCO_3 ratio.
7. **If the clinical picture of the patient does not correlate with the ABG do not hesitate to repeat it before taking drastic measures like intubation !**

Notes

Section IV

How to Interpret an ABG Report

Summary

Read
What is obvious on the ABG report

1. SaO_2
2. HCO_3^- and BE
3. PaO_2
4. $PaCO_2$
5. pH

<u>*MUST read*</u>
What is <u>not</u> obvious on the ABG report

6. $A\text{-}aDO_2$

$$A\text{-}a\ DO_2 = PaO_2 - PaCO_2 - \frac{PaCO_2}{4}$$

SaO_2 v/s PaO_2

PaO_2	SaO_2
40	75
55	88
59	89
60	90
80	95
100	97
140	99
150	99.9

PULSE OXIMETRY

$$SpO_2 = \frac{Oxy\ Hb}{OxyHb + DeoxyHb} \times 100$$

$$SpO_2 = \frac{OxyHb}{Oxy\ Hb + Deoxy\ Hb + CO\ Hb + Meth\ Hb} \times 100$$

Partial pressure of a gas = *Atmospheric pressure (dry)* × *that gas in atmosphere*

PiO_2 = (760 - *Water vapor*) × 0.21
pressure

At sea level water vapor pressure is 47

PiO_2 = 760 - 47 × 0.21
= 713 × 0.21 = 150

Oxygen Content of Whole Blood or CaO_2

$$CaO_2 = (Hb \times 1.34 \times SaO_2) + 0.003 \times PaO_2$$

e.g. (14x1.34x0.99) + 0.003x100
= 18.57 + 0.3 = 18.87 ml

$$pH = Constant\ K \times \frac{log\ Paco_2}{log\ HCO_3}$$

(pH is negative log of H+ concentration)

Relation of pH to H+ ion concentration

(1). $H+ = K \times \dfrac{PaCO_2}{HCO_3}$

$= 24 \times \dfrac{PaCO_2}{HCO_3}$

(2). Change in pH   = Change in H^+ ion
by 0.1   concentration by 20%

Change in pH   =   Change in H^+
by 0.1   concentration by 20%

pH	H^+ ion concentration
7.0	**100**
7.1	80
7.2	64
7.3	50
7.4	**40**
7.5	30
7.6	24
7.7	20

NORMAL RANGES

	Normal Range	Mean
pH	7.35 to 7.45	7.40
$PaCO_2$	35 to 45	40
HCO_3	22 to 28	24

pH of 7.4 corresponds to H+ of 40 mmol

pH less than 7.35 means acidosis
pH more than 7.45 means alkalosis

If Metabolic acidosis look for Anion gap

1. AGMA - Anion gap is high
2. NAGMA - Normal anion gap

If anion gap metabolic acidosis look for Osmolal Gap

Osmolal gap = Measured - Calculated
                 Osmolality   Osmolality

Calculated osmolality = 2 Na + $\frac{Glucose}{18}$ + $\frac{BUN}{2.8}$

Measured osmolality = Calculated osmolality +
                      Osmolality due to other
                      osmotically active substances
                      like alcohols or mannitol

$$ANION \quad GAP = Na - (Cl + HCO_3)$$
An In-vivo phenomenon
(In real life there is no anion gap)

Causes of high Anion Gap 1.Endogenous anions
2.Exogenous anions

Endogenous anions :
Cardiorespiratory failure - Lactate
Renal failure - Organic acids SO4, PO4
Diabetes mellitus   - Keto acids
Starvation   - Keto acids
Anaerobic metabolism   - Lactate
e.g. sepsis, seizure

Exogenous anions :
Salicylates   -Salicylic acid
Ethanol   - Keto and lactic acid
Methanol   - Formic acid
Ethylene glycol - Glycolic and oxalic acids
Paraldehyde

Common poisonings, Anion Gap and Serum Osmolality

Ethanol   : Drinking alcohol
Methanol   : Industrial alcohol
Ethylene glycol   : Wind shield fluidor antifreeze in cars
Isopropyl alcohol : rubbing alcohol used in hospitals
Salicylates   : Many over the counter analgesics

	Anion gap	*Serum osmolality*
Salicylates	*Increased*	*Not increased*
Isopropyl alcohol	*Not increased*	*Increased*

Non Anion Gap Metabolic Acidosis
(Rise in chloride compensates for HCO_3 loss)

Sites of Bicarbonate loss

1. Gastrointestinal
2. Urinary

Causes of Gastrointestianl HCO_3 loss

- Diarrhea
- Small bowel fistula
- Ileostomy
- Uretrosigmoidostomy
- Ileal ureter

Causes of Urinary HCO_3 loss

- Renal tubular acidosis
- Acetazolamide therapy
- Chronic urinary obstruction

Usual picture in various types of renal tubular acidosis

		Urine pH	Serum K+
Distal	RTA I	> 5.5	Low
Proximal	RTAII	< 5.5	Low
	RTA IV	<5.5	High

Metabolic Alkalosis - Look for Urine Chloride

Urine chloride <15 meq/l - chloride responsive
Urine chloride > 15 meq/l - chloride resistant

Chloride Responsive Metabolic Alkalosis

- *Vomiting*
- *Continuous nasogastric aspiration*
- *Volume contracted states*
- *Diuretics*

Chloride Resistant Metabolic Alkalosis

- *Hypercortisolism*
- *Hyperaldosteronism*
- *Sodium bicarbonate therapy*
- *Severe renal artery stenosis*

Remember about $PaCO_2$

*Respiratory rate alone does not tell about
hypoventilation or hyperventilation*

*In patients prone to retain carbon dioxide start oxygen
in lowest possible concentrations wth a close watch on
PaO_2, $PaCO_2$ and breathing pattern*

INDEX

Most of these terms are mentioned on more than one page.
Here those pages are mentioned where they are mentioned in some detail.

Burns - p. 34

ANUP RESEARCH AND MULTIMEDIA LP

OTHER PUBLICATIONS -

ARTERIAL BLOOD GAS ANALYSIS MADE EASY
ISBN 0965708373

MEDICAL SPANISH MADE EASY
ISBN 0965708306

ABG CARD
ISBN 0965708314

PULMONARY FUNCTION TESTS MADE EASY
ISBN 0965708365

**UNCLE ANUP'S BEDTIME STORIES
WITH A MORAL**
ISBN 0965708330

ROMANTIC POETRY
ISBN 0965708322

RELATIVITY OF MORALITY
ISBN NOT YET ASSIGNED

MATRIX CUBE ORGANIZATIONS
ISBN NOT YET ASSIGNED

SHAAYARI (HINDI AND URDU POETRY)
ISBN NOT YET ASSIGNED

DOLPHINS AND SHARKS
ISBN NOT YET ASSIGNED

WHY MEETINGS FAIL
ISBN NOT YET ASSIGNED

ABG SLIDE SHOW (ISBN TO BE ASSIGNED)